Leon Chaitow is a leanaturopathy and acupuncture, who has lectured widely in the United Kingdom, Europe, Australia and the United States of America, and is a senior lecturer at the University of Westminster, London. He practices at the Hale Clinic, London and is the bestselling author of a wide range of health guides.

**Other titles in this series:**

*Arthritis*
*Asthma and Hayfever*
*Diverticulitis*
*Hiatus Hernia*
*High Blood Pressure*
*Prostate Problems*
*Stomach Ulcers*
*Tinnitus*

# Thorsons Natural Health

## Skin Problems

Safe alternatives without drugs

LEON CHAITOW

**Thorsons**
*An Imprint of* HarperCollins*Publishers*

Thorsons
An Imprint of HarperCollins*Publishers*
77–85 Fulham Palace Road,
Hammersmith, London W6 8JB

First published by Thorsons 1987
This revised edition 1998
1 3 5 7 9 10 8 6 4 2

© Leon Chaitow 1987, 1998

Leon Chaitow asserts the moral right to
be identified as the author of this work

A catalogue record for this book
is available from the British Library

ISBN 0 7225 3593 7

Printed and bound in Great Britain by
Caledonian International Book Manufacturing Ltd, Glasgow

All rights reserved. No part of this publication may be
reproduced, stored in a retrieval system, or transmitted,
in any form or by any means, electronic, mechanical,
photocopying, recording or otherwise, without the prior
permission of the publishers.

# Contents

Note to Reader vii

**Chapter 1** The Skin and Health 1
**Chapter 2** The Skin and its Functions 8
**Chapter 3** Sun and Skin 21
**Chapter 4** The Skin in Health and Disease 29
**Chapter 5** Diseases of the Skin (including Eczema) 41
**Chapter 6** Psoriasis, Acne and Other Skin Problems 54
**Chapter 7** Hydrotherapy and Clay 84
**Chapter 8** Diet and Skin Problems 90
**Chapter 9** Stress and Skin 116

Index 130

# Note to Reader

While the author of this work has made every effort to ensure that the information contained in this book is as accurate and up to date as possible at the time of publication, medical and pharmaceutical knowledge is constantly changing and the application of it to particular circumstances depends on many factors. Therefore it is recommended that readers always consult a qualified medical specialist for individual advice. This book should not be used as an alternative to seeking specialist medical advice, which should be sought before any action is taken. The author and publishers cannot be held responsible for any errors and omissions that may be found in the text, or any actions that may be taken by a reader as a result of any reliance on the information contained in the text, which is taken entirely at the reader's own risk.

# 1
# The Skin and Health

There is no common root cause which links the many different forms of skin problems. They may relate to local irritation or infection, to nutrient deficiencies and toxicities, to complex systemic conditions of which the state of the skin is but a side issue, or even to allergic reactions. It is obvious therefore that advice on self-treatment will vary according to the cause of the problem.

Certain conditions will require nutritional correction. In others there might be emotional or psychological aspects, and in many there is evidence of sensitivity or allergy relating to foods or substances in the environment with which the person is in contact directly, or indirectly, such as chemicals, cosmetics, metals, air pollution, etc. In order to provide self-help it is necessary to differentiate between these background causes rather than to concentrate on the obvious symptom.

Natural methods of healing call for a certain underlying attention to lifestyle and nutrition as well as to stress and emotional factors, in order to ensure the removal, as far as possible, of those elements which are working against overall good health. This is true whatever the symptoms. Although desirable changes to the diet may not always 'cure' a particular condition, they will help the body to cope with whatever is wrong.

Therefore a set of general modifications will be suggested which should be assumed to apply to almost all conditions. On the other hand there are certain specific suggestions which apply to particular problems.

## Self-healing at Work

It is assumed that there is a constant self-healing tendency at work within the body. This assumption is easily demonstrated and understood if we realize that all healing occurs without conscious effort, as long as there are no circumstances which prevent this.

When the body defends itself a part of the process involves changes in its function, which we call symptoms. The most obvious example is the change which takes place when anyone is infected with a microorganism and develops a high temperature. This is a symptom not a disease. The raised temperature indicates that the body is at work defending itself against the activities of the bacteria, virus, etc.

*The Skin and Health*

A common reaction at such a time is to treat the symptom, that is to get rid of the temperature. Of course, this would be in complete disregard of the fact that such action would stop the defence mechanism from functioning. The temperature could be made to come down to normal (with aspirin, etc.) but this would be the exact opposite of what the innate intelligence of the body wanted. Its aim is to destroy the invading bug and to restore normality. At that time the temperature would appropriately return to normal on its own.

A far more sensible action in such a situation would be to support the defence mechanisms of the body by reducing food intake, increasing fluid intake, moderate rest, and the taking of helpful nutrients such as vitamin C.

This example illustrates that it is important not to treat the symptoms alone. They are themselves often examples of a self-healing process the suppression of which, by whatever form of treatment we undertake, interrupts the natural healing process.

## Skin as an Organ of Cleansing

The skin, as we shall see, is an important organ of elimination and cleansing of the body and some conditions are no more than evidence of the body doing its self-healing job efficiently. To suppress nature's effort, without regard to the real needs of the body, may cause more problems than are solved. Greater effect would be forthcoming by offering real help to the body, by encouraging in certain instances greater elimination – perhaps using clay compresses or hydrotherapy – whilst at the same time correcting the underlying causes which provoked the body to indulge in a particular form of self-cleansing in the first place.

Certainly there is no harm in doing everything possible to reduce those unpleasant symptoms which may be part of the cleansing process. In relation to skin problems, for example, there may be excessive itching or unsightly blemishes, which can be eased safely without interrupting healing. Such symptomatic treatment should never be at the expense of the overall health of the body, nor in any way impair the healing process.

## Skin as an Organ

We tend to think of the skin as an envelope inside which everything else happens, but in fact the organ of the skin is of profound importance to the overall economy of the body.

It has specific and important functions, which relate to the elimination of waste products, the balance of internal temperature, the control of the body fluid levels and protection from external irritants as well as other more subtle functions.

## The Skin and Health

Because the skin is called upon to carry out many functions it is vulnerable to changes in the individual's general health. There are very few conditions which do not in some manner reflect themselves in the skin, for example, changes in tone, colour, moistness or dryness, etc.

Anyone who is unwell will be aware that changes take place in their overall or local skin condition. It may become drier, more flakey, oily or sweaty; or maybe more wrinkled, less elastic and prone to irritation and inflammatory symptoms, including itchiness.

The skin is a mirror of the internal condition of the body, and the many signs of what is happening are evident to those who pay close attention to its state of health. In the Orient a remarkably accurate system of diagnosis exists, which is based upon the texture, colour and odour of the skin. Many clues to internal status are clear to the observant eye (and nose).

## Underlying conditions

The advice in this book will mainly be related to improving the underlying conditions which have allowed, or provoked, whatever skin condition is being manifested.

Because skin diseases are often the outcome of dysfunction within other systems of the body, it is to these areas that we shall look, rather than simply treating the obvious signs.

## Skin Problems

Few curative agents exist for skin problems, but there are a great many ways of helping skin conditions. Ultimately 'cure' derives from the removal of the causes, which often lie in the person's body or environment.

The skin is no exception to the self-healing tendency which supports us constantly. Anyone who has cut himself can testify to this. A cut results, all other factors being equal, in healing and repair. This leaves, at most, a scar. If we remember that the skin is a major body organ with interconnections to all other aspects of the body (digestive, respiratory, circulatory functions, etc.) then we can appreciate that its own problems often relate to underlying imbalances and dysfunctions which must receive attention before skin health can return.

Our initial intention is to examine the true nature of the skin, in terms of its structure and function, so that we may better understand its problems. This will also aid our understanding of the reasons for particular forms of therapy.

Ultimately we must be aware that healing is the prerogative of the body and anything which we do to support this function should:

(a) be supportive of the body's natural tendency towards repair and normality;
(b) cause no further harm to the body;
(c) take account of underlying causes, whether these

## The Skin and Health

relate to diet, emotions, stress, exposure to irritants and toxic factors, etc.

Whatever we may add in terms of symptomatic relief should keep these objectives in mind if we are to avoid the dangers of merely palliating, without getting to grips with causes.

# 2
# The Skin and its Functions

The structure of the skin is well known, but its functions are less widely understood. The various roles played by the skin may be divided into those which are protective; those which relate to the reception of nerve impulses and the registering of sensations such as temperature for transmission by nerves; the absorption and excretion of liquids and oils; the formation of vitamin D and the regulation of the body's temperature. We will consider these roles later.

First we shall familiarize ourselves with the way in which the skin is constructed. There are two main layers of skin, known as the corium, or true skin, and the epidermis, or cuticle layer.

## The Corium

This deeper skin layer of the corium lies above a layer of subcutaneous fat, which allows the skin to be able to move freely over the underlying structures. The fat deposits of the body are of varying thicknesses in different areas, and of course in different people. The corium is largely made up of connective tissue and constitutes the main part of the structure of the skin. There are numerous blood vessels in this layer, as well as hair follicles and glands for the production of sweat and sebum (sebaceous glands). There are also lymphatic drainage structures in the corium layer.

## The Epidermis

The corium layer is attached to the layer above it, the epidermis, via numerous projections called papillae. These fit into corresponding depressions in the epidermis. Thus the two layers are bound together in a manner which prevents their shearing apart.

The papillae are richly supplied with blood vessels.

Between the epidermis and the corium there is a layer of cells called the basal layer, from which the cells of the epidermis are renewed almost constantly.

Hair follicles penetrate the corium and the epithelium (epidermis) with the root of the hair being contained in papillary projections right down into the subcutaneous tissues (subcutaneous means literally 'under the skin').

There are tiny strands of plain muscle connected to the hair roots, known as arrectores pilorum, which make the hair rise when this is called for.

The sebaceous glands secrete sebum, an oily or waxy substance which lubricates the surface of the skin. These glands open mainly into hair follicles, but some open directly onto the surface of the skin.

The sweat glands are often constructed in the form of coiled tubes and pass the sweat along ducts onto the surface of the skin, where evaporation occurs, thus influencing the temperature of the body. So we have, overlying the corium, the epithelium or epidermis (the cuticle layer) over the entire surface of the body, and which is continuous with the mucous membranes, which cover the lips, nostrils, anus and vagina, as well as the respiratory and digestive tracts.

## Cells

The shape of the cells of the basal layer of the epithelium, which is in contact with the corium, are cube-like and the layer of cells above these are polygonal and contain most of the pigmentation of the skin. The very top of the epithelium is a horny layer of dead skin cells, which are flattened, and which rub off continuously, to be replaced by the multiplication of the lower cells.

*The Skin and its Functions*

## Nerve endings

The nerve endings and blood vessels of the skin are very important. Pain fibres are usually found in the deeper layers of the corium, whereas those which register delicate touch sensations, and heat and cold, are found in both the corium and the epidermis.

The skin may be thought of as a major organ of sense. Indeed more information passes to the brain via the skin than is received from all the other organs of sense combined.

There is a constant feedback to the central nervous system and the brain as to temperature, pressure, stretch and other palpable sensations, from millions of receptors on the surface of the body. This barrage of information enables the controlling mechanisms of the body to make multiple choices as to the needs for action or change, in response to the environment.

It is possible for this facility to be used in the treatment of many conditions, and the practices of acupressure, acupuncture and many forms of massage and manual therapy, as well as hydrotherapy, utilize the skin surface and its amazing nerve supply for this purpose.

One of the most efficient methods of tranquillizing someone is to place them into a 'neutral bath' containing water which is the same temperature as the body. This has a profoundly soothing, indeed almost hypnotic, effect because it allows the millions of temperature receptors in the skin to cease sending information.

If the temperature of the body and its outer environment is constant, this calls for no response from the body, and deep relaxation occurs. This illustrates just how strong an influence the sensory receptors of the skin can have.

## The Blood Vessels

The blood vessels which supply nutrients and oxygen to the tissues of the body, and which drain away used blood, are found in the corium layer, and not in the epidermis itself.

The skin of an average adult covers approximately 18 square metres, and is about .3cm thick. The outer layer is made up mainly of keratin substance which, when it thickens, is recognizable as a callus formation. This comprises thick dry and dead tissue.

The skin is largely, but not totally, impervious to penetration by bacteria and chemicals from outside the body. This is certainly true in ideal conditions, but when factors alter the quality and efficiency of the skin structures, penetration is sometimes possible.

The acidity of the sweat which is produced in the skin also helps to minimize the chances of bacterial growth there.

## Sebum

The production of sebum is most important. It helps to protect and lubricate the structures of the skin and thus prevents excessive dryness.

Sebum is produced where fine hairs grow, so there are no sebaceous glands on the palms of the hands or soles of the feet.

Each hair follicle is attached to a fine muscle which causes the gland to express the sebum, when compressed or contracted. With alterations of temperature the glands therefore alter their production.

The glands are not uniformly active and many influences impinge on their production of sebum, including excessive tension in associated muscles. The condition of acne is often connected with these glands and their production of sebum.

## Sweat Glands

Sweat glands exude water and organic salts.

Some 2.5 million of these tiny glands exist in the average body, and are plentifully present on the soles of the feet and palms of the hands.

Some are constructed as straight tubes; others have a more tortuous structure, something like a corkscrew. The largest sweat glands are found under the arms and in the groin, where they are particularly active.

Each sweat gland has a nervous supply and a connection with the blood supply of the area.

Modified sweat glands produce the waxy material found in the ears.

The lipids excreted via the skin keep it smooth, being natural emollients. If the pores become blocked this can impede excretion and add to the chances of local infection developing, resulting in 'spots'.

Skin which is dry is not lacking in water, but rather in lipids, and therefore becomes scaly.

## Antiperspirant Sprays

It is considered that the sebaceous gland excretions help to contain and minimize the activity of bacteria and fungi on the skin, and this factor should lead to caution in the indiscriminate use of deodorant and antiperspirant sprays.

It can be shown that if the skin is impeded in its excretory efforts, the body temperature rises, and in many cases the breath becomes foul, as elimination is switched to the lungs.

The control of sebum and sweat production is closely linked to hormone activity, as well as nervous system influence. The lymphatic structures, which are found in the skin, are concerned with the removal of waste material. The influence which we may bring to bear on the lymphatic and circulatory structures, via the use of hydrotherapy (water treatment) for example, is very strong, and can be of great value in dealing with many skin problems.

Thus in considering the skin, we should realize we are dealing with a very complex structure, which protects us from the outer world as well as providing us with an interface with it, so that we may register all sorts of alterations in our environment. The skin is both a shield and a source of information for the body. It is an organ which can be used to eliminate unwanted materials from the body, alter temperature and form vital vitamins.

## Temperature Adjustment

One of the most important functions of the skin is its relation to temperature adjustment. The average temperature in man is around 37°C (98.4F). This is held more or less constant, under an amazing number of variable conditions, indicating a sensitive system of control. The degree of efficiency with which the body succeeds in this can be used as a measure of how healthy an individual is. There exists a tendency towards normal at all times, and the mechanisms which the body employs to achieve balance and normality, in all its functions, are called homoeostatic functions.

## Homoeostasis

Homoeostatic functions have a reasonably wide range, within which they can still be regarded as being inside normal limits. The wider the variations and swings away from normal, the greater the degree of stress is being placed on the body.

For example, it is known that there is a normal level of sugar in the bloodstream. This will vary depending upon activity or emotional factors (which lower it) and eating (which raises it). In a healthy individual, on a balanced diet, the variations in extremes between the highest and lowest levels in any one day will be modest.

When the diet is unbalanced however, with a high sugar intake, or where great stress factors are at work, the variations between the highest and the lowest recorded blood sugar levels will be great. At a certain point in time the body ceases to be able to maintain balance and ill-health becomes apparent.

Thus, in the example of blood sugar, a diabetic situation (high blood sugar) and hypoglycaemia (low blood sugar) may be manifested. This is when diseases and symptoms first become apparent. Earlier signs of wide swings within the 'normal' ranges of blood sugar would have been an indication that problems were going to develop.

Homoeostasis represents the body's effort to maintain the many variables, in all the multitude of functions and processes operating in the body, somewhere around normal, in the face of myriad factors in the internal and external environment which are imposing strains and demands on the system.

In the case of the maintenance of normal body temperature, the function of the skin is of paramount importance, since it has the ability, in a variety of ways (but principally involving the sweat glands) to control the internal temperature. The wider the range between normal sweat production and the often apparent copious production, in some people, the greater the homoeostatic effort of the body.

Thus we might recognize that anyone with excessive sweat production is calling upon their body to cope with demands which may ultimately manifest in the form of illness or dysfunction. The range of function from 'normal average' to 'over-active' and on to 'feverish active', and ultimately to collapse and disease is observable in a study of people under different conditions, and in the same person under different conditions.

Let us try to understand how the function of control of body temperature operates.

## What Produces and Controls Temperature?

The temperature of the body is a result of two elements – the amount of heat generated by metabolism and activity, and the amount of heat lost via normal channels. Under normal conditions any additional heat produced is taken care of by increased heat loss.

## Skin Problems

Heat is produced by muscular activity and by the activity of the organs such as the liver. When the body is cold the action of shivering is an attempt to raise the temperature by movement of the muscles. Hormonal activity (e.g. the thyroid) can also produce heat generation.

As food is processed for use within the body, it causes a degree of temperature increase via oxidation. The body also gains heat from the external environment, as well as generating its own in response to various activities, its metabolic function, etc.

Heat loss may occur via the skin, or by the warming of air which is exhaled by the lungs. This latter facility is more important to animals than it is to humans since few animals have sweat glands.

The skin becomes warm because it is so richly supplied with blood vessels to the corium. Heat is also conducted to the corium via the underlying muscles, although this is minimized by the presence of subcutaneous fat deposits which are poor conductors of heat.

Once heat reaches the skin it is lost to the outside via radiation, convection and evaporation. The latter is the most efficient method and is largely affected by air humidity.

Radiation of heat is increased by the blood vessels in the corium becoming dilated so that the skin flushes. As more warm blood passes through these vessels heat is lost.

*The Skin and its Functions*

Convection takes place when air comes into contact with the skin. This is more likely when no clothes are covering the area, and is most obvious when cool air is passing over the skin, as in exposure to a breeze or fan.

Evaporation occurs as liquid (sweat) passes through the pores, and is greater when the air is relatively dry.

There is evidence that heat regulation is controlled by a centre in the brain, and is therefore under nervous system guidance.

## Fever

Fever often commences with the body's attempt to conserve heat, and may involve shivering and restlessness. There should be no attempt to depress such an innate attempt on the part of the body's defence mechanism to heal itself, of which vital function fever production is often a part.

Problems relating to the skin can result from interference with any of the heat-control mechanisms described, which are among the most important functions of the skin. The fluid loss via perspiration is a medium which the body may choose to eliminate unwanted materials. Evidence of this excretion through the skin of sometimes toxic materials indicates that this channel is of considerable importance to the body's economy, and relieves other more obvious routes (e.g. kidneys). Even under normal conditions many acid wastes are passed through the skin for elimination, together with the perspiration.

Various skin problems often arise following interference with normal skin function: e.g. overuse of undesirable cleansing agents contained in some soaps, or excessive sebum production which blocks channels of excretion, or a build-up of excessive layers of keratin because of lack of vitamin A.

## Sunlight

Sunlight, so vital to life, is also a major skin irritant when excessively exposed to this.

Degeneration of the elastic tissue of the skin results, and dry inelastic wrinkled skin structures eventually become obvious. The ultraviolet content of sunlight may produce alterations in the cells with potential dangers which we shall examine.

There is a relationship between skin ageing and skin diseases, including cancer of the skin, and the excessive exposure to sunlight of this natural barrier inside which we live.

# 3
# Sun and Skin

Professor Albert Kligman, an expert on skin health, has said: 'Skin care should begin at six months of age. We are the only animal put on this earth naked. The sun, wind, rain and so forth do 90 per cent of the damage. To prevent (early) ageing we've got to prevent the environment having direct access to our skin.'

This is perhaps an extreme view but the facts are that the sun can be a great hazard to skin health, with serious repercussions.

At least 10 per cent of the new patients seen by dermatologists have skin cancer of one type or another. It is certain that a combination of ultraviolet light from the sun and an inability to produce enough melanin (which tans and thus protects us from penetration of the sun's rays) is a major cause of this. Among the important indicators of this are the following:

## Skin Problems

- There is a higher incidence of skin cancer in sunny countries.
- There is more skin cancer in fair-skinned than in dark-skinned people.
- There is a low incidence of skin cancer in people who have black or yellow skin.
- There is far higher incidence in people who work out of doors.
- The rise in incidence of skin cancer over the last half-century parallels the increased involvement of the population with outdoor activities.
- The fairer the skin and the greater the exposure to sun, the shorter the period of incubation before skin cancers appear. In countries such as Australia and South Africa as well as the southern and western US, young people of 20 years of age may display the first signs of malignant skin disease.

In the UK this may not be shown until individuals reach their forties. Of the patients with skin cancer in the UK, fully one-third of those over the age of 50 are directly related to sun exposure, and of those over 75 years of age one-half the skin cancers are sun-induced.

People who burn, rather than tan, when exposed to the sun, or those who have relatives with sun-induced skin cancer, should ensure that children of the family are thoroughly conditioned to protect themselves from the sun. They are advised to do the following:

- Avoid direct sunlight wherever possible.
- Wear adequate covering when in the sun.
- Use sunscreens on those areas exposed to the sun.
- Avoid holidays which involve sunshine exposure.
- Make sure that employment is indoors and that sunny countries are not chosen to work or live in.

Skin cancers are largely preventable by avoidance of the irritant, ultraviolet light.

If you are in any doubt about a skin wart or nodule which has altered its behaviour by changing shape, size, colour (dark brown, black or blue) or which has started itching, become inflamed, ulcerated, developed crusting or is bleeding without cause, then seek advice from a medical practitioner forthwith. Early attention is essential in skin cancer, which is easily contained at the outset.

## Sun Protection Creams and Lotions

There are now many lotions and creams available with varying degrees of efficiency in screening the skin from the sun. They are identified by a number which is known as the SPF (sun protection factor). The number indicates the percentage of filtering agents in the product.

There are two types of filter used. Sunscreens filter the UV (ultraviolet) rays, but still allow tanning to take place. Sunblocks contain opaque pigments and absorb or reflect all UV rays and thus do not allow tanning to take place.

The higher the SPF number in any product the more protection the skin gets from burning rays. Those with the higher numbers in any product range will contain sunblock.

There is, unfortunately, no standardized numbering method amongst the various competing brands of SPF creams. Take care and seek advice from a good pharmacist, in order to establish which SPF factor offers the protection you require.

## Professor Kligman's Advice

There should be a concerted attempt from a very young age to protect the skin from the ravages of the sun and weather (see Professor Kligman's advice at the beginning of this chapter).

He advocates a programme for any type of skin but which is particularly suitable for dry-skinned individuals. The regular use of a lubricating gel such as petrolatum (Vaseline for example) is a basic strategy. Take a fair-sized 'blob' of this onto the fingertips and massage into the clean skin with gentle circular movements for a minute or so. Then use a tissue to remove all the excess.

The essence of this skin treatment is that you cannot get it all off. You can remove sufficient so that the skin

## Sun and Skin

feels pleasant to touch, but a certain amount will remain lodged in the tiny crevices of the skin and will act as a lubricant. The Professor advises a daily application.

The regular use of sunblocks every morning is also recommended, with extra applications if outdoor activities are frequent.

'No one has a suntan without injury. If you must tan do so safely. This means wearing a sunblock not just in the sun but at all times, even in winter. Only expose your body in the early morning or late day sun, and don't tan your face.'

Professor Kligman's suggestion is based on a lifetime's experience of disease and death resulting from skin cancer, and is accompanied by the information that by the age of 20 three-quarters of all damage to the skin has already occurred in most people. The effects, though, may not be seen until about the age of 40.

The extreme view taken by this expert is obviously designed to provoke at least some response, and to increase awareness of the well-known, but often ignored, hazards of sunlight.

Remember the basic advice. When you are sunbathing use a protective cream which lessens the UV rays' chances of burning the skin. If you are fair-skinned or have a family history of skin cancer, then use sunblocks as well.

*Skin Problems*

Everyone would be well advised to heed the advice never to sunbathe other than early or late in the day, and never at midday.

Ageing of the skin as a result of excessive sunlight involves the development of solar elastosis, which is characterized by a flabby, dry, leathery feel to the skin, deep wrinkling, and loss of surface markings. This is the 'weathered' look, which has become old before its time, in response to being burned and heated excessively. There is no way of restoring such skin to normal; prevention is the only logical approach.

These changes take place in the DNA and protein strands in the cells, which develop cross-linkages and thus lose their elasticity, very much like rubber when it becomes weathered, fragile, perished and impoverished. The prospect of having skin which behaves like tired elastic should alert everyone to the foolhardiness of excessive sunbathing.

Since tanning relates to vanity and a desire to improve appearance the almost inevitable end result of a leathery wrinkled skin can be the exact opposite of the effect desired.

## Photodermatosis

Many people develop a sun-related rash. This is differentiated, as a rule, from other rashes because it seldom appears in places where the sun is unlikely to reach, such as under the chin and nose, the upper eyelids and behind the ears.

There are variations of this type of light sensitivity and apart from general health enhancement, as recommended later, the avoidance of direct sunlight via the use of appropriate sunscreens and keeping out of the sun is recommended.

General health, including nutritional, improvements have often made such sensitivities less pronounced and have been shown at times to remove the sensitivity altogether.

The following factors can make photosensitivity more pronounced:

(a) the use of antihistamines and drugs such as thiazides, frusemide, tetracycline, griseofulvin, phenothiazines, chloroquine, etc. Also sulphonamide drugs which have been used systemically or on the skin;
(b) certain cosmetic preparations, including musk *ambrette*, eosin in lipstick, quinine in hair tonic, bergamot oil in eau-de-Cologne;
(c) soap, deodorant and shampoo contents, such as hexachloraphene and bithionol;
(d) contact with certain plants such as hogweed, parsnip, cow parsley, carrot, celery, lime and chrysanthemum;

## Skin Problems

(e) various dyes including red and yellow used in tattoos.

Use of, or contact with any of the above (and there are more) should be investigated if a rash develops commonly after exposure to sunlight. This may be safely soothed with camomile lotion.

# 4
# The Skin in Health and Disease

The skin is often provided with an opportunity to act as a diagnostic medium, in that many diseases produce signs apparent in the skin, although it may not itself be involved.

Before we consider those changes in the skin which may become apparent when health conditions are less than good in other body systems, we shall look at the nature of healthy skin and of protective measures relating to it.

In good health the skin is supple and has a visible sheen. 'Just like a baby's skin' is what we should aim for, even in later life. This quality relates both to the natural lubricants of the skin, as well as to the regular reduction of the surface layer of dead cells by natural friction. When these surface cells remain unstimulated, and thick layers accumulate, a dullness will be found in the skin quality. Skin should be elastic and soft; any other texture, even in the elderly, is unnatural and relates to changes and causes of which we will touch upon.

The ageing process leads to a slow loss of elasticity, but this can, to a large extent, be minimized by appropriate careful nutrition and skin hygiene.

## Vitamin D

Up to three-quarters of the body's vitamin D requirements is manufactured in the skin. This is the product of an interaction between sunlight and the skin.

Calcium metabolism in the body is dependent upon vitamin D presence, an important element in preserving a sound bone structure. In babies the amount of vitamin D which can be produced by the skin of the cheeks alone is prodigious.

The fact that sunlight is so important to body health does not mean that we should easily expose ourselves to this hazard, as already discussed. Short periods of exposure are all that are needed, say 30 to 60 minutes daily, depending upon the intensity of the sun. We do not need to lie and cook ourselves; even sitting in the shade, outdoors or by an open window, allows for adequate exposure.

As with so many things in life the fact that something is good for us, or even essential in moderate amounts, does not mean that unlimited amounts will be even better. On the contrary, just as a short cold shower is toning, a long cold immersion is harmful. So with sunshine – a little is good and even essential to health; too much is damaging and dangerous.

Ultraviolet light from the sun is an antibiotic. However, excessive amounts will not only destroy harmful bacteria which might be present, but also useful ones which live on the skin of most people. These maintain a healthy environment by destroying undesirable, unwanted micro-organisms.

Thus skin health is essentially a matter of balance – a desirable diet, which we will discuss later; good hygiene (which does not mean over-washing, for this removes the natural lubricants); adequate, but not excessive, sunshine; desirable deodorants which do not block the skin (when deodorants are necessary, that is); and adequate friction and stimulus of the skin to remove the dead outer layer. These are some of the main prerequisites of a healthy skin.

## Air Baths

Exposure to air is more beneficial than exposure to the sun. A period during which the naked, or nearly naked, body is in the fresh air, if temperature allows, is beneficial to skin health. It has a toning effect on the circulation, with additional benefits being derived from stimulating this function further by briskly rubbing the skin surface with a rough towel, a loofah, or even the hands.

If outdoor exposure is impossible then the same procedure, in an airy room, suitably warmed, is recommended. The air bath is a habit which should be encouraged in children especially.

Colds and coughs are far less frequent in those who do this, since their response to changes in temperature, which may sometimes trigger a cold, is less erratic. The skin, thus toned, becomes capable of dealing with variations in temperature more efficiently. It also becomes healthier in appearance because of the friction effect.

## Helping Elimination

Because the skin is an organ of elimination and great quantities of perspiration, and acompanying salts and acids, pass through it daily, there is every need to ensure that the efficiency of the process is maintained, as well as employing adequate means of ensuring the cleansing of the pores and the skin itself.

Heavy and unsuitable clothing, which fails to allow for adequate evaporation of perspiration is undesirable. Underclothing should allow for a degree of ventilation, and therefore natural fibres such as cotton, and string vest-type materials, are preferable to allow air movement. The greater the envelope of clothing, the greater the burden placed upon the lungs which have to take over some of the skin's functions when it is restricted in this way.

Antiperspirants are a similar burden upon the lungs and should be avoided.

If the skin is kept toned by use of air baths and friction and is not overburdened with clothing, there will be less danger of colds developing and the skin will carry out its eliminative functions more efficiently. Regular active (aerobic type) exercise will further enhance skin function.

## Bathing

Regular bathing is necessary in order to prevent the accumulation of surface deposits of excreted salts and acid wastes. Showers are probably more desirable than baths and should be taken at moderate temperatures, not too hot. A final few seconds under cold or cool water is stimulating to the skin and circulation, especially if followed by a brisk towelling friction.

Choose your soap carefully. Your pharmacist will advise on which soaps most perfectly maintain the skin's acidity at its correct level. Many soaps destroy this and can cause problems. Some soaps remove too much of the natural lubricants of the skin and are also undesirable. Perfumed soaps are often the most guilty in this respect, and simple soaps designed for sensitive skins should be sought.

A daily bath or shower ensures cleanliness and skin toning if this advice is taken, and is an integral part of any skin-health programme. This of course assumes that there is no good reason for not having a bath or shower, which is sometimes the case.

## Fat

Skin health will vary with the degree of underlying fatty tissue which, if excessive, leads to consequent loss of elasticity, sensitivity and good colour. Circulation is often impaired in the skin when fat is carried to excess. Dietary measures, also exercise and toning procedures such as skin friction, are often the answer to such problems, with nutrition as the main element.

As we will see later, vitamins A, C, B complex, F and other nutrients such as zinc, as well as essential fatty acids, are all vital for sound healthy skin function.

Undesirable foods, especially those devitalized by processing (white flour, sugar products, etc.), saturated fats (fried food, most animal fats, etc.) and the destructive effects of alcohol and smoking, are probably the greatest irrirants in this respect.

Attention to these factors will ensure, all other things being equal, a healthy skin. This is a double asset in helping overall health, via elimination and temperature control, as well as providing an attractive outer covering for the body.

## Skin Changes in Ill-health

When skin changes occur it is important to discover whether or not the problem is related only to the skin or whether it is associated with a systemic condition.

A very loose skin, which can easily be lifted in folds, is an indication of a major loss of weight.

A harsh greasy skin may often (though not always) accompany tuberculosis.

An overactive thyroid gland usually causes a general moistness to the skin, especially on the palms of the hands. In contrast, when the thyroid is underactive, in the condition known as myxoedema, the skin is extremely dry.

A condition which produces a hard thickened skin texture is called scleroderma. Fortunately, this is extremely rare.

In people of African descent (mainly) there is a disease called icthyosis in which a scaling occurs, particularly on the legs. This is a congenital condition.

A watery condition under the skin (generalized oedema) may accompany kidney disease, heart disease and diabetes.

The colour of the skin may be related to different conditions. For example an extreme paleness is noted

## Skin Problems

in anaemia, although not all pale people are anaemic, but simply lack a rich supply of superficial blood vessels. True anaemia would be accompanied by a paleness of the mucous membranes.

If the skin is reddened to an unusual degree, it may indicate scarlet fever, or of course recent prolonged sunbathing.

In some blood conditions, such as polycythaemia vera, there is a reddish-purple colour noted in the skin of both the hands and face.

A yellowish tinge, of a lemon hue, is seen in pernicious anaemia, and sometimes in secondary anaemia.

An orange colour is sometimes seen in diabetes, especially on the palms. It may also be accompanied by orange-coloured nodules on the skin which relate to a high cholesterol content of the blood.

Jaundice also produces yellowish discoloration. This colour change may also tend towards a greenish or brownish tinge and is best observed in daylight.

Such changes should not be confused with carotinaemia, which may occur in individuals who have consumed excessive amounts of carrots or other orange-coloured vegetables. In this condition the sclera of the eyes do not change to orange, as they would in jaundice.

A bluish change in the skin colour is called cyanosis and relates to oxygen starvation. This might occur for a number of reasons, including cardiac disease and pneumonia. The ears and tip of the nose are usually

## The Skin in Health and Disease

the first places to be affected. In congenital changes of this sort, where the heart is involved, the lips will be blue. Cyanosis may also result from poisoning by certain drugs and chemicals.

Poisoning by silver salts may result in a grey-blue discolouration of the skin (argyria) which, although permanent, is apparently harmless.

In Addison's disease there is a striking brownish or bronze-like discolouration, which is also seen in a condition known as haemochromatosis. Patients with Addison's disease are usually tired and have very low blood pressure, a consequence of the exhaustion or non-functioning of the adrenal glands which characterize this problem.

A number of other skin changes should be mentioned in passing related to systemic conditions.

The medical use of drugs such as sulphonamides and antibiotics frequently produces skin eruptions.

Many conditions result in small reddish papules under the skin. There is usually an extravasation of blood in such spots, as in a blood blister, and depending upon their size they are called by different names. Spots of this type which do not disappear when pressure is applied to them are called purpura. When they are very small indeed, like a pinhead, they are petechiae, and when large they are known as ecchymoses.

These are different from the red spots found in conditions such as typhoid fever, 'rose spots', which do disappear when pressed, for they are caused by increased blood supply under the skin, rather than blood which has escaped into the skin structures.

Purpura are seen in some blood diseases and vitamin deficiencies such as scurvy (vitamin C deficiency). In cerebrospinal meningitis they are a common finding, hence its other name of 'spotted fever'. Petechiae are found in many conditions including leukaemia, inflammation of the heart muscle, and aplastic anaemia; also less frequently in forms of cancer, TB and kidney disease.

When the capillaries (small blood vessels) are fragile, a condition noted when vitamin K is deficient, petechiae often occur after even slight bumps and knocks.

Small reddish spots, which on close examination show as tiny blood vessels radiating from a central site, are known as 'spider naevi' and suggest liver disease, often cirrhosis. They are also noted in deficiency conditions and in pregnancy.

In some people there is a striking instability of the skin circulation, which allows for a condition known as dermatographism, or autographism. In this it is possible, by lightly stroking the skin, to produce weals which remain for some time. In bygone days these were called 'witch's marks' and the unlucky individual so affected often perished at the stake.

None of the above conditions would respond to local treatment, and in many cases unless underlying, often serious, pathology were dealt with there would be little chance of improvement. This highlights the need for identification of causes, before the institution of anything other than palliative treatment.

There is no reason not to improve skin problems by self-help methods, and indeed much can be done by simple measures whilst underlying problems are dealt with.

There are a number of skin complaints which originate other than in the skin structure itself, as well as some which are purely local in origin and manifestation.

## Smoking and the Skin

The skin is a visible sign of our general state of health.

It has been shown that smokers can now be identified by their facial skin texture and wrinkles – almost infallibly, by simple scrutiny of the face or by photograph.

Characteristic lines radiating from the mouth and deep vertical lines on the cheeks or upper lips are frequently noted, as is a loss of good colour and a generalized grey or yellow tint to the skin. The increased wrinkling which occurs in smokers is caused by damage to the oxygen supply and an increase in the activity of so-called 'free radicals' in the body, which promote premature ageing of the tissues. Not only the skin is affected of course, but this is the most visible sign of such damage.

*Skin Problems*

# Alcohol and the Skin

Similar changes, not as dramatically visible perhaps, occur with the increased use of alcohol (and, to a lesser extent, of refined foods).

Few skin conditions relate only to the skin, even in the case of skin infections. Most are part of a larger problem and by examining the various conditions we will see how the interaction takes place between the skin and the general health of the body.

# 5
# Diseases of the Skin (including Eczema)

Before considering individual conditions there are some patterns of skin complaints which commonly occur.

Red scaly eruptions are medically termed erythemato-squamous dermatopathies. Among these are eczemas, superficial fungal diseases, psoriasis, pityriasis rosea, secondary syphilis, discoid lupus erythematosus and lichen planus. Not all of these are suitable for self-treatment and we will only consider those which are.

Each of the above conditions may be divided into further subgroups. For example, there are many types of eczema: notably atopic eczema, contact eczema, seborrhoeic eczema, discoid eczema, stasis eczema and chronic hand and foot eczema, among others. It should be emphasized that underlying many of these apparently different forms of skin disease, may lie very similar causative factors.

The word dermatitis is often used interchangeably with eczema. For practical purposes the word eczema is used where causes arise within the individual, and the word dermatitis is used where the causes appear to arise from outside the body. (Contact dermatitis, for example, may result from skin contact with a metal such as nickel.)

Raised weals on the skin occur in a variety of conditions including urticaria, erythema-multiforme and a nodular version called erythema nodosum.

Skin infections include furuncles (boils), sycosis barbae, carbuncles, axillary hidradenitis and impetigo, as well as acne (which is sometimes associated with massive bacterial infection).

The term infection is used in these conditions because there is involvement of pathogenic micro-organisms. This is not the same as saying that the conditions are caused by micro-organisms, and the frequent medical concentration on annihilating the bacteria or viral factors neglects the underlying conditions which are often the cause of bacterial proliferation. In self-help methods it is important to consider deeper causes than are obvious, if long-term relief is aimed for.

A variety of skin conditions relate to viral activity, including warts, verrucae and herpes infections.

*Diseases of the Skin (including Eczema)*

Parasites may also occur in the skin, such as ringworm (a fungal parasite), athletes' foot and scabies (caused by a mite), and lice.

Acne is one of the most troublesome of all skin conditions, especially for the adolescent. Aspects of this condition relate to sebaceous gland activity, hormonal factors and infection.

Some less common conditions such as pemphigus vulgaris, dermatitis herpetiformis and rosecea will be touched on.

## Eczema (Atopic Dermatitis)

Eczema is a chronic itchy, inflammatory skin condition in which the skin is very dry. The lesions may be seen as patches of reddened, sometimes weeping areas, scaling, with small vesicles present in the skin itself. There is sometimes lichenification in which additional pigment is noted in plaques of thickened skin, with accentuated furrows. Scratching and rubbing leads to this lichenification, especially in areas such as the elbow, wrist and knee creases.

There is frequently a family history of eczema. The patient has to contend not only with the discomfort of the condition, but also often with severe emotional distress in consequence of its unsightly nature.

Ignorance of the true nature of the ailment often leads to feelings of guilt or 'uncleanliness', which are totally unwarranted. There is no danger of spreading the disease to others as it is in no sense an infection. Thus children should not be left out of sports or other contact activities for fear of contagion. Unfortunately the degree of unpleasantness endured by victims of eczema, from the unfeeling and thoughtless behaviour of others, can cause severe emotional damage.

Family life can also be strained because of the sleepless nights associated with children thus affected, scratching and restless as they frequently are.

Eczema must be differentiated from other similar conditions, for example, fungal infections such as scabies or psoriasis (*see Chapter 6*), pemphigoid and vitiligo, etc.

Medical diagnosis should always be established before trying to treat the condition.

Where the cause lies outside the body (exogenous eczema) there may be specific irritants or allergic contacts which require identification. There is also the chance that the sensitivity is to light (so-called photo-allergic or phototoxic eczema). In such cases the individual would be aware of the connection and the lesions would be sited only where light reaches the skin.

## Development of Eczema

The sequence of development noted in acute eczema is of an initial redness of the skin; the formation of

## Diseases of the Skin (including Eczema)

vesicles may progress to form either blisters, or may rupture to release fluid which forms a crust. This is called 'weeping' eczema.

Chronic forms of the condition show a redness and scaling of the skin, due to lack of cohesion in the outer layers. Fissures appear and pigmentary changes occur. Secondary to this, as a result of scratching and rubbing, holes may be gouged in the skin by the nails, and lichenification takes place in which thickened skin and exaggerated skin markings appear. Infection can result from such irritation.

The main irritants which have been noted as being involved in such conditions include detergents, alkalis, solvents and bleaches. The sufferer may also become allergic to some quite innocuous substances such as nickel in costume jewellery or rubber (gloves, etc.).

The history of the condition is the only way of accurately assessing the cause, since the appearance is always the same. Testing with contacts of different substances may identify irritants (patch testing) and improve the condition when the suspicious substances are removed. But even if an irritant is found and removed, the explanation as to why this particular person is sensitive to this substance remains unanswered. It is the underlying cause of such sensitivity (which may of course be inherited) which should receive attention, as well as the removal of obvious irritants.

In atopic eczema the skin is usually dry and pale, and there is almost always some family connection or history of the condition. Itching and lichenification is frequent and occurs more commonly on the cheeks of babies, the elbows, knees, wrists and ankles of children and the palms and sides of the fingers in adults.

Seborrhoeic eczema is usually noted in adults and results in reddish-brown, greasy, scaling areas, rather than vesicles. The scalp, eyebrows, paranasal areas, the arms, chest and between the shoulder blades are the usual sites.

When seborrhoeic eczema affects infants it starts in the nappy region and spreads to other body creases. Sometimes the scalp is affected (cradle cap) and it may progress to become atopic eczema, or disappear on its own.

An unusual variant occurs which has oval or round plaques scattered over the trunk and limbs. These are characterized by weeping and vesicles. This is called nummular or discoid eczema.

## Medical Treatment

The treatment of eczema by medical means usually involves the use of hormone creams, known as topical steroids. The side-effects of these are seriously worth considering. Local skin thinning occurs, as does easy bruising, and a tendency towards subsequent poor wound healing. The constant use of these drugs

*Diseases of the Skin (including Eczema)*

involves the serious risk of damage to adrenal gland function and the induction of other serious skin diseases, such as acne, rosacea, folliculitis and tinea.

## Self-help Treatment

Ideally treatment of eczema should always involve the removal of identifiable irritants such as detergents, antiseptics, bubble baths, soaps, etc. Non-soap cleansers are available from pharmacists (aqueous cream or emulsifying ointment) and should be used in the place of conventional soaps.

Itching may be eased by the use of certain herbal substances such as aloe vera juice.

Atopic dermatitis (eczema) is very common and affects about one person in 20. It is known that certain changes in the body occur in individuals with atopic eczema and that these often relate to hypersensitivity towards certain substances and foods. Many of those affected initially by this condition go on to develop allergic rhinitis (characterized by a stuffed or runny nose, much of the time) or asthma, and almost all such patients improve on what is known as an 'elimination diet'.

This aspect of natural self-help treatment of skin problems is common to many folk, and a diet which suits one person will not necessarily suit another. See Chapter 8 for further information on diets for skin disease.

## Food Allergies

There are some common foods which appear to upset the majority of cases, and these include a generalized sensitivity to milk (especially cow's milk). Even soya milk may irritate many individuals. It is worth noting that breast-fed infants are less likely to develop eczema than bottle-fed infants. If breast-fed infants do develop the condition, it often occurs at weaning when new foods are being introduced, often of cereal origin.

Breast-feeding mothers may consume milk, or other substances, which then pass on to the baby, so it behoves them to take special care of their diets, particularly if their children are showing signs of eczema.

The following outward signs may be noted when allergic conditions are operating:

- dark circles under the eyes
- chronic fatigue
- a horizontal crease in the lower eyelid
- chronic swollen glands, especially under the ears and jaw
- a chronic tendency to accumulate fluid, unrelated to other factors such as monthly periods.

The commonest foods to avoid if seeking a quick solution of a possible food allergy, without the admittedly lengthy procedures which are called for in elimination diets, are the following: wheat and all cereal products;

## Diseases of the Skin (including Eczema)

corn; soyabeans and their products; cow's milk and all its products; eggs; all food preservatives and additives.

There is a greater awareness of the immune system (the defence system of the body) because of the publicity attached to AIDS. When allergies exist the immune system is reacting abnormally and requires assistance.

## Dietary Supplements

In all cases of atopic eczema, therefore, a number of specific nutrients are suggested in order to support the immune function. These include selenium, zinc and vitamin B complex. Vitamins A and E are also called for, and details of the quantities suggested will be found in Chapter 8.

The extract of cold water fish known as EPA (eicosapentaenoic acid) is another very useful dietary aid which boosts the presence of essential fatty acids in the body, an important factor in eczematous conditions.

In order to reduce the aggravating inflammatory skin processes, often involving the substance histamine, it is suggested that the nutrient quercetin be taken. This is an anti-inflammatory bioflavonoid substance which occurs in nature, often in combination with vitamin C, in plants. The bioflavonoids are known to be helpful in reducing the permeability of the fine capillaries and thus improving skin function.

An extract of the pineapple plant, the enzyme bromelain, is another powerful anti-inflammatory agent with a damping effect on substances called kinins, which along with histamines take part in inflammatory processes such as eczema.

There are certain other sources of essential fatty acids, such as the plant evening primrose, the oil of which has been found to be useful in allergies in general, and eczema in particular.

## Bowel Health

In eczema, as in many other skin complaints, the function of the bowel and the health of the flora of the bowel are usually poor. The flora is composed of the helpful (and sometimes less than helpful) bacteria which live inside all of us, and which not only assist digestion but also manufacture essential substances for health.

Attention to this function is important, since problems with digestion lead to problems with absorption and transportation of nutrients. This has direct bearing on the health of the skin.

It is suggested that a powerful *Lactobacillus acidophilus* powder should be taken by anyone with a skin problem, for a period of not less than three months and ideally six. These *acidophilus* bacteria repopulate the bowel with friendly bacteria and help to control the activity of undesirable ones which might have gained a foothold. This is commonly the case in allergic conditions and in eczema.

*Diseases of the Skin (including Eczema)*

Some forms of strong *acidophilus* powder are free of all milk products and are suitable for anyone who is milk sensitive. For those not sensitive to milk there are other strong sources.

If an expert in nutrition is consulted, tests involving digestive and bowel function may be undertaken, also assessment of the possible involvement of the fungus Candida albicans. However, where self-help methods are being employed it is best to stick to advice which is safe and simple, and this includes the use of one or other of the suggested cultures of bacteria for the bowel.

## Thyroid Test

In order to assess whether or not there might be an underactive or overactive thyroid involved in a skin problem, take the underarm temperature for 10 minutes on three successive mornings before getting out of bed.

If the temperature averages under 36.5°C (97.8°F), the thyroid is probably underactive and a course of thyroid extract may be called for. Such tendencies commonly accompany eczema. This would require medical prescription. If the temperature averages over 36.0°C (98.2°F) the thyroid may be over-active and medical advice should be sought.

## Skin Problems

## Local Treatment

Local treatment of itching skin may be helped by the use of zinc oxide cream or lotion. Greasy preparations should not be used as they block the pores. Rough-textured materials and undue sweating should be avoided.

A useful cleansing action for the liver and bowels is green clay powder, consumed in the form of a drink (see page 84 for instructions). If a bath is taken it should not be a lengthy one, and any eczematous areas which are to be wetted should be covered first with a paste made from green clay and olive oil. This will protect the area and prevent irritation by the water.

Clay has marvellous properties as a cleansing and healing agent and can be used internally or externally.

One of the most potent of all plant extracts for eczematous areas is the juice of aloe vera. This desert plant has astounding healing properties. The recommendation for its use in both eczema and psoriasis is unqualified. One or two tablespoons of the juice should be consumed daily in water, and applications of the juice should be made to the affected areas at least twice daily.

If the skin is dry, aloe vera ointment may be more suitable because it has an astringent action. A mixture of aloe vera and pure almond oil is an effective dressing for dry eczema.

*Diseases of the Skin (including Eczema)*

It is essential for anyone with a condition such as eczema to reduce stress and anxiety levels, and relaxation exercises, together with an accompanying stress-reduction programme, should be considered (*see Chapter 9*).

## Summary

- Avoid all known irritants, chemicals and rough materials.
- Eliminate undesirable foods and pay attention to eating correctly and to bowel function. Institute elimination and/or rotation diets and seek out and eliminate food allergens.
- Support immune function with listed nutrients.
- Employ bioflavonoids (quercetin) and bromelain as suggested.
- Use local topical dressing as suggested (clay, aloe vera, etc.).
- Introduce stress-reducing methods as suggested.

Note:
In this and many other skin conditions, symptoms may appear worse for a short period after instituting self-help methods. This is quite normal.

# 6
# Psoriasis, Acne and Other Skin Problems

Psoriasis appears to be an inherited condition. It is characterized by itchy, scaly red patches, usually beginning with tiny scale-like lesions which join together and which, when severe, may disfigure much of the body surface.

Psoriasis is rarer in non-whites and affects men and women equally, usually starting to manifest itself between the ages of 15 and 30. Psoriasis may, however, appear at any age, from infancy in the nappy (diaper) areas, to old age, even after a lifetime free of the condition.

There are many variations in this condition both in appearance and intensity. The commonest patterns are:

- Scaly red patches, especially on knees and elbows.

- Dandruff: scaliness on the scalp (large scales) with well-defined patches and red skin under the patches, typically at the edge of the hairline. There are often scales clinging to the hair, which may be thinning. Such signs may indicate that this is not ordinary dandruff but psoriasis. *(See also 'Seborrhoeic Dermatitis', page 76.)*
- Patches of plaque formation on the creases behind the knees and in other flexures and creases of the body such as the spaces between the toes, the groin and above the anus.
- Nail dystrophy may occur in which large pits appear on the surface of the nail, or the end of the nail becomes obviously discoloured, often with a yellowish tinge. They take on the appearance of 'oil drop' stippling.
- There might be a development of a widespread rash of scaly red discs up to 1 cm in diameter. This may only last for a month or so and is more likely in people under the age of 30. It is often accompanied by tonsillitis (this is called guttate psoriasis).
- People with inflammatory diseases such as arthritis have a greater tendency towards psoriasis.

Other variations exist, but these are the commonest forms of this sometimes disfiguring and usually distressing condition.

The rate of replication of cells in psoriasis is amazing and exceeds normal cell division by 1,000 times, an even faster rate than is found in cancer. Even the rate of division of skin cells in the normal skin of people with psoriasis is some 2½ times faster than usual.

One of the safest methods of keeping the condition under control for many sufferers is regular exposure to natural sunlight or artificial ultraviolet light (UVL), for two or three short periods weekly. In a very few people, however, this makes the condition worse.

The longwave UVL is more effective than short UVL in helping psoriasis, but is also more dangerous, especially to fair-skinned individuals (*see Chapter 3*). Medical treatment attempts to increase the effect of the UVL by giving light-sensitizing drugs such as methoxy-psoralen, before exposure to sunlight or a lamp. The amount of sunlight should be minimal, since any sunburn (in the same way as any skin injury) would be likely to turn to psoriasis. This approach is effective in roughly half of all psoriasis patients.

It is interesting that in Egyptian times an extract of a weed growing by the Nile was used in exactly this manner, with apparent success, in psoriasis cases. The extract of the weed is the base of the modern drug which sensitizes the body area to light.

The longwave UVL needed is also similar to the light found in regions such as Egypt. This has made the area of the Dead Sea a favourite for people with psoriasis to go to for therapy.

## Hydrotherapy at Home

A similar home treatment can be obtained by using either Epsom salts (about 1 kg) and sea salt (about 500 g) in a warm but not hot bath; 'Dead Sea mud' and salt, which is now widely exported from both Israel and Jordan (the Dead Sea lies between these neighbouring countries), can be purchased and used in a home bath, as can various 'Dead Sea' skin preparations, designed for psoriasis and other skin conditions.

## Other Approaches

Other medical approaches include the use of tar applications, hormone creams, radiotherapy and other drug applications. All these have varying degrees of danger and side-effects attached to their use, with radiotherapy and steroids (hormones) being potentially the most hazardous.

Although they do not 'cause' the condition, there exist a number of triggers to psoriasis, such as infection with streptococcus (of the tonsils, for example) and the use of certain drugs (e.g. lithium, some antimalarial drugs and corticosteroids) and also, less frequently, anxiety. Most people who develop psoriasis,

## Skin Problems

however, appear to develop the condition with no apparent cause.

Spontaneous recovery is not uncommon, with remissions being unpredictable, short or long term. In some cases, unfortunately, there appears to be an unremitting state in which nothing appears to help. In such cases the natural approaches suggested should be used consistently for a few months to assess their effects.

# Natural Self-treatment

General advice which may help – if applicable – is as follows:

- If the individual with psoriasis is overweight, losing some of the excess may help considerably.
- Reducing or completely cutting out alcohol can be very helpful, as virtually any alcohol consumption is harmful for psoriasis.
- Adequate rest, sleep, exercise and fresh air should be ensured, as well as taking care of dietary habits, as discussed below and in Chapter 8.
- It is important to avoid letting the skin become dry. Using safe products (such as an unguentum cream, from a pharmacy) to maintain skin moisture levels is therefore very important.
- Scratching or peeling the dry skin from psoriasis lesions should be avoided at all costs.

## Psoriasis, Acne and Other Skin Problems

## Diet

Nutritional excellence is called for in dealing with psoriasis naturally. There is no doubt at all that, as in eczema and so many other skin conditions, intestinal health is a key factor in psoriasis. The diet for general skin health should be followed (*see Chapter 8*) and there are also certain basic nutrients which require extra emphasis in the diet, and/or by supplementation, as outlined below.

One of the main findings as to what is happening regarding diet and psoriasis is that protein digestion in particular is somehow faulty. There seems to be an excessive degree of toxicity in the bowel – with the accumulation of abnormally high levels of toxic amino acids (protein particles) such as putrescine and cadavarine in the gut. These are far less likely to be found if a low-fat, low-sugar, vegetarian diet is followed. There are also a number of herbal and nutritional supplement strategies which can help to reduce the toxic levels in the intestinal tract (*see below*).

With psoriasis liver function is also often found to not be as efficient as it should be, perhaps as a result of this major detoxification organ having to deal with the excessive levels of toxins from the bowel.

It is for these reasons that fats, alcohol and sugars – in particular – should be kept to a minimum in the diet. There are also certain tactics which can help with protein digestion and bowel toxicity.

## Better Protein Digestion and Bowel Health

The *vitamin A* suggested later in the section about supplementation for psoriasis helps to retard the formation of undesirable toxic compounds, as does the herb *Hydrastis canandensis* (Goldenseal), and this may help if taken regularly for some months.

Recently there has been a great deal of interest in the benefits for psoriasis patients in taking a few drops daily of *oil of oregano*. This must be obtained from a reputable source, and taken in a little warm water for best effects. Oregano, as with many aromatic herbs, has powerful detoxification (and antifungal) effects.

Far more important is to improve protein digestion; this can be assisted by taking *proteolytic enzymes* (enzymes which digest protein and which are normally sufficiently produced by the pancreas but which may be in short supply in those suffering from psoriasis). It is suggested that:

- Before a protein meal: 1 teaspoonful in warm water of a herbal mixture called Swedish Bitters. Helps to promote digestive function and better protein digestion.
- 500 mg of a pineapple derivative called bromelain (available from health food stores) should be taken with each meal where protein is a main constituent.
- 2 to 4 teaspoons of aqueous extract of the plant sarsparilla is recommended. This is found to bind

those toxins in the bowel which have been associated with psoriasis.

Supplementation with a combination of *Lactobacillus acidophilus* and *Bifidobacteria* (available either individually or combined) is highly recommended twice daily as a means of boosting the friendly bacteria colonies in the bowels. These act to detoxify endotoxins, which contribute towards psoriasis.

The herb *silymarin* (milk thistle) aids the liver in its detoxification tasks. Available as liquid or capsules from health stores. Different brands will have their own recommended dosage, but it is felt that between 100 and 200 milligrams (mg) of the herb daily should be taken to assist liver function.

*Sulphur* is a major cleansing and detoxifying element which is found in abundance in eggs (yolks) and in such vegetables as onion, garlic, mustard and horseradish. From this the body makes certain amino acids, particularly cysteine and methionine, both of which play major detoxifying roles in the body. These may be taken regularly (see dosage in Chapter 8) along with sulphur-rich foods – an egg or two daily (free-range) and frequent use of onions, garlic and mustard greens in cooking will serve as good sources. Another source of sulphur is old-fashioned molasses, which also has a laxative effect.

To help with bowel toxicity and immune system support, the herb *Hydrastis canandensis* (Goldenseal) is suggested. This is assisted by herbs such as *Echinacea* and *Berberine*, which have similar influences (immune-enhancement, antifungal, antibiotic, etc.). *Hydrastis* and *Berberine* (and often *Echinacea*) can be found in combination in many formulations, often further combined with zinc and vitamin E.

Also try to find a supplier of oregano oil and use this as described earlier in this chapter. Failing this, make a tea of regular dried oregano and drink this at least once daily.

Ask at good health food stores for information regarding these herbs, as taking them regularly is recommended for general health, bowel health, immune support and psoriasis.

## General Nutritional Assistance

As with so much medical treatment, the tactics used in psoriasis usually aim at symptom control with little attempt to deal with underlying causes. Natural self-help methods must do so or will also fail to achieve any real progress.

The condition of psoriasis is complex and space does not allow for a full explanation of the reasons for the various nutrient suggestions which are made. Suffice to say that they are all aimed at dealing with aspects of the biochemical problems which underlie this skin disease and so help to restore normality.

*Vitamin $B_6$* (pyridoxine) and the element *zinc* act together in many body processes and are important in skin health. These are recommended for psoriasis in dosages of 50 to 100 mg daily of $B_6$, and 15 to 30 mg daily of zinc. (A form of zinc which is readily absorbed is important; one such kind is zinc orotate. A 100-mg zinc orotate tablet would contain about 15 mg of zinc.)

*Vitamin A* should be taken to assist in preventing the build-up of bowel endotoxins – 10,000 to 20,000 iu daily is recommended.

Just as zinc is needed, so is additional *calcium* – 500 mg daily is suggested as a regular supplement to the diet.

As in eczema, the antioxidant bioflavonoid *quercetin* (quarter teaspoon of powdered form several times daily) is suggested as an anti-inflammatory agent together with *vitamin E* (200 to 400 iu daily) which should be taken with the mineral *selenium* (found in garlic in rich supplies) – 50 to 200 micrograms (mcg) daily.

It is also suggested that oil derived from fish, (*eicosapentaenoic acid – EPA*) and either the oil of the *evening primrose* plant (500 to 1,000 mg daily) or a dessertspoonful of cold-pressed *flax seed oil* (linseed) be taken daily as a source of essential fatty acids.

*Vitamin C* is contraindicated in psoriasis, and should not be supplemented in high doses. A general health supplementation of this important protective vitamin, of 500 mg daily, would not, however, cause any problems.

## Detoxification

Therapeutic fasting and a balanced vegetarian diet – as outlined in Chapter 8 – will also help to cleanse the bowel effectively.

At least 40 per cent of individuals with psoriasis report that a major stressful event occurred a month or less before the onset of their condition; this leads to the suggestion that stress-reduction methods, as outlined in Chapter 9, could be helpful.

The basic approach to psoriasis treatment should include detoxification strategies as well as supplementation as indicated.

Specifically there should be a limit on the intake of sugars and animal fats as well as vegetable oils in any quantity, apart from those recommended. A high fibre intake is essential to keep bowel function healthy and to aid in binding and eliminating endotoxins from the bowel.

Any food allergy should be dealt with by elimination and rotation diets (*see Chapter 8*).

Sunlight should be used in moderation, no more than one hour per day. Local treatment may be helpful with oil of evening primrose or zinc oxide ointment directly onto the skin lesions.

## Acne

Over 50 per cent of young people are affected by acne, but it is severe in only about 3 per cent of boys and to a lesser extent in girls. Unfortunately many adults suffer acne throughout their lives, often intermittently (for example around period time) but sometimes persistently.

It occurs only in areas of skin where there are actively functioning sebaceous glands, especially on the face and upper trunk, and does not appear at all in individuals who have no male sex hormones (eunuchs); thus it is known to be dependent on hormonal influences, or at least greatly influenced by these.

When acne occurs there is almost always an increased production of sebum in the skin of the area affected. The more sebum, the worse the acne. Inflammation is caused by the presence of bacterial infection in the sebum (*Propionibacterium acnes*), which causes it to break down into irritating fatty acids.

Blackheads are caused by the presence of a dark plug which blocks the sebaceous duct or a hair follicle. This plug is made of the pigment melanin and causes a build-up of sebum behind the plug, eventually resulting in pustular formation which erupts on to the surface (*acne vulgaris*).

If the breakthrough of the pus to the skin does not happen, a closed form of acne occurs (*acne conglobata*) which may spread into underlying skin layers with possible cyst or abscess formation, resulting in a lumpy appearance to the skin.

The psychological and emotional effects of unsightly acne, especially during the difficult teenage years when appearance is so important, makes this a condition worth taking seriously, even though in overall health terms it does no real harm.

There are a number of different forms of acne, as in all skin conditions.

## Teenage Acne

A typical picture is of the face or upper trunk being affected by angry reddened spots, which may develop into pustules or papules. The condition often commences at puberty and persists throughout adolescence, with periodic flare-ups. Eruptions may be sparse or very heavy.

At puberty (or just before), hormone production increases, particularly androgen hormones such as testosterone. One of the effects of this is to cause an increase in the production of sebum and of the substance keratin. In young skin the pores may be smaller than can cope with the extra production of these substances, leading to the blockages described above, with subsequent bacterial involvement (these bacteria are normally present on everyone's skin) leading to pus formation and 'spots' or cysts.

## Psoriasis, Acne and Other Skin Problems

One of the reasons for blockage of pores is the accumulation of dead cells; this highlights the need for regular washing and use of cleansing agents to remove these cells and any accumulated dirt.

In some cases acne is actually the result of exposure to industrial chemicals such as cutting oils, diesel oil and other mineral oils derived from petrochemicals which add to the likelihood of the pores becoming clogged. In such cases, as in all acne, good hygiene is important (regular washing and clean clothing) as well as use of a well-formulated barrier cream. Other professions affected include those operating with tar and pitch, as well as those exposed to insecticides, herbicides and wood preservatives.

It is safe to say that most teenage acne starts for reasons over which the person affected has little control, such as the particular amount of sebum being produced in response to hormonal changes, together with the size of pores. However, hygienic factors can usually be controlled, and if acne continues there is a great deal that can be done to eliminate or control it.

Picking or squeezing spots is always unwise as this prolongs their duration and often results in scars.

Before looking at strategies to help control acne, we need to examine another group of people who are regularly affected by acne: women.

## Acne in Women

Eruptions often (but not always) relate to period times, as hormonal changes occur. Use of the contraceptive pill is often suggested as a means of controlling severe acne in many women, however there is evidence that in some cases it is the Pill itself that is making matters worse – either due to a further disturbance of hormonal levels (the Pill is a hormone medication) or because of interference which the Pill produces in the normal bacterial population living inside our bodies (discussed later in this section).

Cosmetics affect many women, especially if they are excessively oily. Great care is needed in finding products which are acceptable. Perhaps avoiding their use altogether for a time is a wise strategy.

If you have acne and you use cosmetics, the following 'rules' may be helpful:

- Do not use any oil-based cosmetics, or soap, or cleansing agents on areas where acne is present or where it commonly appears.
- Look for products which actually state that they are free of oil – although this will not guarantee that the product will not contain chemicals which may be irritant to particular skins, since cosmetics contain hundreds of different chemical substances.
- Also avoid cosmetics which contain any wax, so read the labels carefully. Unfortunately the word

'hypoallergenic' does not mean that a product is safe; nor does the phrase 'ideal for oily skin' – or some such use of words.

- Take care, on areas prone to acne, to use only light cosmetic cover – such as a very light application of a non-oily (gel or dry powder) blusher. Any heavy cover cosmetic will simply add to the likelihood of pores becoming blocked, with all that this leads to. If a base is being used ensure it is a liquid, oil-free one, and ideally dilute it slightly with water.
- Take extra care regarding moisturizers as these often add to acne problems rather than helping the skin. You can prove this for yourself by using such a product on one half of your face only for a while and judging the results.
- Despite the advice to 'avoid all oil-based products' there is one enormous exception, and that relates to Tea Tree oil products, about which more will be found later in this section. Tea Tree oil is a remarkable natural anti-acne product, but it needs to be used correctly for best results.

## Skin-cleansing Strategies

Skin care

- A thorough twice-daily (morning and evening) cleansing of the skin with calendula or a solution containing sulphur is suggested.
- Also apply Tea Tree gel or solution (15%) at least twice daily.
- Tea Tree oil (*Melaleuca alternifolia*) is an oil derived from an Australian shrub which has powerful and safe antibacterial and antiviral effects. When it is applied on the skin to pus-containing areas (wounds as well as acne spots) it is particularly useful. Care needs to be taken to use it in a diluted form as it can irritate the skin if used neat. Many products are available, including an excellent 'pimple gel' (Blackmores) which deals with acne outbreaks very rapidly.
- Use of the cleansers recommended here will help to clear excess sebum and to prevent blockage of the follicles, but it may take several months to get acne under control. Other measures are also necessary – including dietary changes.
- Regular sunshine or UV lamp for 20 minutes daily is helpful in many cases.
- Clay: The use of the natural substance clay on the affected skin area is often extremely helpful. Green

clay should be made into a mud-like consistency and applied to the area several times per week for an hour or more at a time, including use as a face mask. This is soothing, cleansing and highly recommended.

## Medication and Acne

Drugs used to treat acne are often based on vitamin A derivatives. Some side-effects to these are common, including excessive dryness of the skin and flaking, which may be persistent. They need to be used under expert guidance and only in severe acne conditions, because of the potential side-effects.

The long-term taking of antibiotics to destroy the local micro-organisms which take part in the acne process is often successful but carries long-term dangers, such as provoking the spread of fungal colonies which inhabit the body (*Candida albicans*, for example, about which more will be found in Chapter 8).

Antibiotics not only attack the harmful bacteria which take part in the development of acne but also destroy 'friendly' ones which control these yeasts. There are many undesirable long-term effects which can follow on from antibiotic usage, not least the damage to the friendly bacteria and the development of resistant strains of bacteria which can be life-threatening. It makes no sense at all to try to improve a cosmetic problem, even if it is causing emotional discomfort, by helping to create the potential for really serious diseases. As we will see below, natural methods are less hazardous and include dietary measures, stress-reduction and also local treatment.

It is of interest that severe acne is often noted in people who later become affected by cardiovascular disease. There seems to be a common nutritional link; excessive consumption of sugars and fats is probably the major factor.

## Natural Self-help Methods

Acne may respond well to exposure to sunlight, but recall the advice given regarding the dangers of over-exposure. Trying to tan your way out of acne will only age your skin more rapidly.

Despite medical opinion being divided on the subject, those involved in nutritional medicine know that diet is a basic factor in acne. Among commonly found associations with severe acne is a degree of bowel stasis and toxaemia, often diet-related (usually a high-sugar, high-fat diet) but also often related to damage done to the bowel flora by antibiotic medication.

## Dietary Strategies

- It is necessary to reduce carbohydrate intake, especially of sugars, and to increase protein intake to adequate levels, not less than 3 oz daily. As with eczema and psoriasis, the health of the bowels is vital, and similar procedures are called for as are discussed earlier in this chapter and in Chapter 5.
- Foods containing *iodine* should be avoided (such as seaweed, which also means kelp tablets) as this aggravates acne.
- Animal fats should be severely restricted because of the harm they do generally as well as the problems they cause in the digestive tract.
- In order to help the body deal better with carbohydrates, an addition of a *chromium supplement* is often needed. This is part of the glucose (sugar) tolerance factor as it relates to acne (400 mcg daily is suggested).
- *Vitamin A* in high doses is helpful but should not be undertaken without supervision and so is not part of a self-help programme.
- *Zinc* is also useful in acne, as in so many other skin problems. It is involved in local hormone activation as well as control of vitamin A activity, wound-healing and tissue regeneration (20 to 40 mg daily is suggested).

## Skin Problems

- Together with zinc, *vitamin B_6* is needed as these work together in many processes. This is especially true if acne is worse before or during a woman's periods. 100 mg daily is suggested.
- *Vitamin E* and *selenium* have an influence on acne and are suggested as regular supplements to the diet. (400 iu of E and 200 mcg of selenium are recommended.)
- Dietary changes are recommended, including *low sugar*, *low fat*, *high fibre* and *protein*, as well as the use of *acidophilus* and the supplemental nutrients mentioned.

## Stress Reduction

In trials on severely affected teenagers in Florida, it was found that regular relaxation exercises reduced the incidence of acne dramatically. Over a three-month period those youngsters using simple relaxation techniques had better overall results than those who had regular medical care. Over a one-year follow-up those who kept the exercises going (15 to 20 minutes a day) maintained their improvement, whereas those who stopped had relapses. Despite this fact, the number of individuals who continued the programme was less than 30 per cent, which indicates that motivation was not adequately encouraged.

## Dermatitis Herpetiformis

This is a pruritic blistering rash found mainly on the limbs of middle-aged white persons (males most commonly). It is a direct result of sensitivity to gluten, a major component of wheat and other grains. Wheat is the greatest irritant and must be eliminated. The use of the B vitamin para amino benzoic acid (PABA) helps to control symptoms. An elimination diet must be used to assess all allergens apart from grains, and those foods involved should then be omitted from the diet (*see Chapter 8*).

## Erythema Multiforme

Symmetrical inflamed, swollen, sometimes papular lesions are present which have the appearance of a target, with a clear centre surrounded by concentric rings of redness.

The back of the hand is a common first site. The lesions are usually found on the arms and legs. It happens more frequently in spring and autumn, and is commonly a response to the use of drugs such as penicillin, sulphonamides and barbiturates. Vaccination may trigger this complaint, and also infection with herpes simplex virus or food allergy.

The taking of *potassium iodide* may be all that is needed to control the problem, but this can cause other skin problems in some cases and should only be undertaken with supervision. Local treatment with *zinc sulphate solution* is suggested if herpes infection is the cause (0.05 per cent solution).

## Seborrhoeic Dermatitis (SD)

SD may be confused with eczema but is far more common. It is a relatively harmless condition but has the potential for causing itching and irritation and being unsightly.

Most adults in industrialized countries suffer from SD at some time, and many all the time. Many skin experts believe that once you have shown signs of SD it will always be present and from time to time will manifest more actively because of changes in circumstances (*see below*).

The word seborrhoeic means 'oily' and of course dermatitis means 'inflammation of the skin'. So the whole name of the condition is one which indicates that there is an oily inflammation of the skin – even if the area feels 'dry' to you. The combination of excessive oil production and activity of bacteria which are a normal part of the skin environment is the cause of SD.

SD involves a combination of itching and flaking – and sometimes reddening of the skin, commonly on the face, around the ears, eyebrows, nasal creases, between the eyebrows, and on the hairline as well as on the chest, arms, legs, armpits, groin and so on.

When it occurs on the scalp itself and falls as flakes, we call it dandruff, although with dandruff there may also be a yeast infection associated with the dermatitis. Anti-dandruff shampoos aim to control these excessive microbial overgrowths and so prevent, or reduce, the condition.

SD develops in many people during puberty and has a definite hormonal connection, with some women finding a link with phases of their menstrual cycle.

The reason that SD is often noticed for the first time at puberty is that special oil-secreting glands in the skin become more active at this time, leading to more oil production and the triggering of an explosion of microbial activity, with seborrhoeic dermatitis as the outcome.

The condition varies a great deal throughout the year, with a decrease after exposure to sunlight, especially during the summer, and an increase of activity in the winter. Other factors which seem to have an impact on the severity of the condition are emotional stress and hygiene.

The first signs of SD usually appear on the scalp and then spread to the hairline, the face and possibly other parts of the body.

SD is not contagious. The micro-organisms involved in the process are always present on your skin throughout life, as mentioned. What happens is that the environmental conditions change, perhaps due to hormonal fluctuations, perhaps due to poor hygiene, perhaps because of stress; dietary deficiencies or excesses or a food intolerance (allergy) often contribute as well. It is usually some such combination of variables which alter the environment in which the micro-organisms live, so triggering a population explosion – with the results already described.

## Treatment

Apart from examining the possibility of food intolerance (*see 'Allergy' in Chapter 8*), certain supplements have been found to assist in treating SD.

1 Biotin – 500 mcg should be taken twice daily (at breakfast and evening meal).
2 Separately from this, 100 mg of vitamin $B_6$ should be taken (say with the midday meal).
3 At the evening meal, a full spectrum B-complex capsule should be taken containing no less than 30 mg of each of the major B vitamins.
4 As with so many skin complaints, extra zinc is called for – 20 to 30 mg a day.
5 A tablespoon (at least) of cold-pressed flaxseed oil should be consumed daily, on cereal, with yogurt, on salad or neat.

## Hygiene

Use of medicated shampoos can be helpful, and it is the scalp which requires the most diligent attention. A safer and more natural product is Tea Tree shampoo, now available from most health stores and many pharmacists. Tea Tree oil shampoo has remarkable properties as an antifungal and antibiotic which does not harm the skin.

The hair and scalp should be shampooed at least three times a week (using medicated or non-medicated shampoo) with the lather allowed to stay on the scalp for a considerable time – up to 10 minutes – before rinsing. A gentle scrubbing of the scalp during the time the lather is in place is helpful, taking care however that the skin is not broken in the process.

Expect the 'flakes' of dandruff to be more abundant at first; this will soon pass.

Use of a diluted (15 per cent) Tea Tree solution on the skin wherever red, flaking skin is present is useful, if you are sure that this is not eczema. If it is eczema, the Tea Tree solution will irritate the patches. Always get a responsible and accurate diagnosis first before trying self-treatment.

# Herpes Infections

The infection of the body by herpes simplex virus can affect the face around the mouth (cold sores), the eyes or the genital regions. In each case the infecting agent is the same and can be spread from one place to another, and to other people, by direct contact. The best method of control is a diet which *increases the intake of lysine* (an amino acid) and *decreases arginine* intake (another amino acid).

This has been found to reduce the ability of the virus to replicate. Lysine-rich foods, which are also low in arginine, include fish, chicken, cheese, beef, beans, brewer's yeast and mung bean sprouts. Those which have a high arginine content and which should be avoided include chocolate, carob, coconut, oats, wholewheat and white flour, peanuts, soybeans and wheatgerm.

Most fruits and vegetables have an excess of lysine over arginine and may therefore be eaten freely. *Vitamin C* has a protective effect on the lysine levels in the body.

A daily lysine supplement of between 300 and 1,200 mg is recommended, along with not less than 1 g of vitamin C.

The homoeopathic remedy *Rhus tox* (6X) has been found to control and reduce further outbreaks of herpes virus. It should be taken three times daily.

## Ringworm

This fungal infection is best treated by raising general body health through optimum eating habits (*see advice in Chapter 8*).

Crushed or sliced garlic may be applied locally to the lesion. This should be bandaged in place and replaced once or twice daily. Garlic is a potent antifungal agent, and this approach has proved to be more effective than antifungal drops.

## Rosacea

This is a strong redness which affects the facial structures and is often disfiguring. Patients with this condition usually have a high level of reaction to stress. They blush and flush easily in response to anxiety, alcohol or spicy food, which should all be avoided as much as possible. *(For stress reduction advice see Chapter 9.)* General nutritional improvements should also be made.

## Sycosis Barbae

Spots appear on the face, not unlike acne, but in this case they occur only in males after puberty and are caused by the bacteria *staphylococcus aureus*. Lesions always have a central hair protruding. Control is possible via hygiene of the skin and dietary changes such as apply to acne.

Removal of the central hair with tweezers will deal with individual spots, but this is a first aid measure only and does not address the underlying condition.

## Summary

We have now considered several common skin problems in detail and others in passing. There are many more, of course, which we have not dealt with, either because they do not lend themselves to self-help methods or because they are part of larger systemic conditions which require more complex attention.

It should be clear, though, that the main elements to recovery from the conditions discussed are similar: dietary factors, sometimes involving allergy and often requiring supplementation; stress reduction, and local therapy using safe substances such as water, aloe vera juice and clay.

Even the nutrients required are the same for quite different conditions: zinc, vitamins A, E, C and some of the B vitamins; essential oils such as EPA and evening primrose; amino acids and, that most important element of all, *acidophilus* for restoring bowel flora health, a factor which cannot be over-emphasized for all skin problems.

## Psoriasis, Acne and Other Skin Problems

In general the use of hydrotherapy and clay treatment to the skin is suggested wherever inflammation is present. Various applications of these safe methods make them applicable in most conditions. Anti-inflammatory nutrients such as quercetin and bromelain are recommended for most inflamed skin problems.

# 7
# Hydrotherapy and Clay

Green clay from France has both healing and detoxifying properties. It is a superb natural product and may be used with complete safety in a variety of ways.

## Internal Use

In order to facilitate cleansing of the digestive tract and the binding of endotoxins which may develop or arrive there, a drink of water in which clay has been dissolved is recommended. A teaspoonful of fine green clay is stirred into a tumblerful of lukewarm water and allowed to stand for at least half an hour before the water is consumed, leaving the sediment in the container. Another way to consume clay beneficially is to make small pellets and bake them in the oven until hard. These may be swallowed a few at a time daily. The clay will dissolve in the bowel and, as with the drink above, will allow small amounts to reach the small and large intestine where it will absorb toxic substances.

## External Use

In cases of skin eruptions clay may be used directly onto the skin surface, where it has a dual role: it soothes inflamed and irritated skin at the same time as drawing out impurities, acids and other toxic substances which may be aggravating the condition. Clay is mixed with water to form a paste and then spread over the skin area where it can be allowed to dry before carefully washing it off after an hour or two.

It may be covered with a bandage and left in place for longer periods, even overnight if desired, to give it more time to do its work. Remove it carefully. Most of the clay may be peeled off in one piece, but if some clings to the skin it may be dabbed free with a solution of aloe vera juice or olive oil, or left to come off in its own time.

Where skin is very dry the clay may be mixed to a paste with pure virgin olive oil and similarly spread over the skin area. Lightly bandage into place and leave for up to 24 hours. Removal should be easier than with the water-based paste. The oil-based paste is unsuitable for conditions where the skin is suffering from an excess of sebum or oil (e.g. acne).

## Hydrotherapy

There is a long history of the beneficial use of water treatment in skin conditions.

For skin which tends to dryness, olive or almond oil should be massaged lightly over the body and into all skin folds, particularly where there is a tendency to flaking, before taking a bath. Use only a safe soap or aqueous cream. If there is any sensitivity or inflammation, pat the body dry, otherwise a brisk rubdown using a dry towel will improve circulation.

A general cleansing and toning effect on the skin may be effective in cases of recurrent boils, carbuncles (multiple boils), or even acne. This may be achieved by use of an *Epsom salt bath*. Dissolve 450–700 g of commercial epsom salt (available from any pharmacy) in a bath of tolerably hot water. No washing takes place. The person lies in the water for 10 to 20 minutes and then after drying should lie on a bed covered with a blanket for an hour or more. Sweating is often profuse after such immersion. As an additional boost to the value of this bath, 250 g of sea salt may be added to the water at the same time. This sort of bath is potentially tiring and should not be undertaken more than twice weekly and not at all if the individual is weak or frail.

## Hydrotherapy and Clay

The result of an Epsom salt bath, on an otherwise healthy individual, will be to stimulate circulation and elimination through the skin. It is not recommended for people with eczema, but may benefit those with psoriasis, acne, boils or carbuncles.

A soothing alternative to this is an *oatmeal bath* wherever there is an irritation of the skin, including eczema or psoriasis. Place 900 g of fine oatmeal in cheesecloth bags and put into the bath as it is run. The water should be luke warm. Lie in the bath and do not attempt to wash, but allow the essence of the oatmeal to lightly bathe the body. The bags may be squeezed periodically to extrude more 'oatmeal juice'. Ten to 15 minutes of this is suggested. This is a soothing treatment rather than a stimulating one such as the Epsom salt bath.

Where you need to treat a skin condition locally, which is inflamed and/or painful, a compress may be used. This is known variously as an *evaporation compress* or *a cold compress*. The affected part is covered with a piece of damp cloth, which retains a good deal of plain cold water. This is left in place for a minute or two and then replaced. The contact with damp, cold material will reduce inflammation.

As a variation on this, wring out the damp material (cotton is ideal), place over the inflamed area and cover with a dry flannel or woollen material. Fix this firmly in place by pinning or bandaging. This produces a

## Skin Problems

sequence in which the initial coolness of the material is warmed by the body heat which is then retained and eventually bakes itself dry. Where there is any attempt to eliminate acids or toxins through the skin this is an effective boost to the body's effort. This sort of compress may be left in place for up to eight hours. The material should be thoroughly washed before re-use, as it will have absorbed toxic wastes.

Where boils or abcesses are discharging or near to discharging their pustular contents, *hot fomentations* are suggested. They are also useful where areas of hardened scales of skin are present. Wring out a piece of woollen cloth in water which is as hot as may be tolerated. Apply immediately to the area and cover with a dry woollen cloth. Leave in place for some minutes until it has cooled off. It should then be replaced. If the skin is dry and scaly, lightly rub with pure olive oil prior to the application. Psoriatic lesions respond well to repeated use of hot fomentations.

*Aloe vera juice* is a superb healing agent with no contraindications. It is of value on any inflamed area and also on wounds. It may be used neat or diluted and as frequently as desired.

Where there is a tendency to scar formation on the skin, for example after a burn, the regular use of the oil of *vitamin E* (found in capsules of vitamin E designed for consumption) is suggested. When rubbed lightly into the affected area it will minimize the inflammation (vitamin E is an antioxidant) and reduce the danger of scar formation. It will also reduce existing scars. Vitamin E creams are available but many have additional substances designed for cosmetic purposes; a capsule of vitamin E oil is preferable.

# 8
# Diet and Skin Problems

There are various dietary factors which can help to normalize and prevent skin problems; some of these have been spelled out in the earlier chapters that dealt with specific skin complaints.

There are general strategies which will help almost any skin complaint, as was proved by some important research conducted by a leading American nutritional expert, Professor E. Cheraskin of the University of Alabama. In an attempt to identify previously unrecognized variables in the genesis of skin disorders, he examined – using interviews and special questionnaires – the dietary and medical histories of over 1,000 doctors and their spouses associated with the University. He found that those individuals who reported one or more skin-related symptoms, as compared with those who reported no skin conditions at all, had a significantly

## Diet and Skin Problems

higher intake of refined carbohydrates (mainly sugars) in their diets. Also when Cheraskin analysed the vitamin C intake of the diets of those people with the fewest skin problems, he found that they were taking significantly more than those people with more skin problems.

The following questions were asked:

- Is your skin very sensitive or tender?
- Do cuts in your skin usually stay open a long time?
- Does your face often become badly flushed?
- Do you sweat a great deal, even in cold weather?
- Are you often bothered by severe itching?
- Does your skin often break out in a rash?
- Are you often troubled with boils?

Over a period of a full year, Cheraskin carefully monitored the two groups, those with few (or no) skin problems and those with several.

He also asked the group with fewest skin problems to increase their intake of vitamin C by a small amount, from an average of around 240 milligrams (mg) daily to 430 mg daily. After one year there were even fewer skin problems reported in the group of people taking the higher vitamin C levels.

These two studies (sugar and skin problems and vitamin C and skin problems) were independent and it is logical to suggest that a combination of high vitamin C intake and low sugar intake would provide the ideal background strategy for general skin health through nutrition.

With many of the skin conditions we have examined there are of course other factors to be taken into account, with allergy being one of the most important.

# Allergy

As we have observed in looking at various skin conditions, there are a number of disorders, ranging from urticaria to eczema, which are related directly to allergy or food sensitivities.

Identification of the foods involved calls for detective work. A number of different detection strategies are outlined here, some less complicated than others.

## Method 1: Complex Elimination Diet

This method is founded on the idea that the main known irritants – based on many years of clinical research by allergy specialists – should be excluded from the diet.

The most prominent allergy-provoking foods are known to be:

- milk and all its by-products such as butter, cheese and yogurt
- cereal products (grains of all sorts including wheat, barley, rye, oats and millet – but not including rice

## Diet and Skin Problems

and buckwheat, which are not grains)
- eggs and all products containing egg
- refined and processed foods and anything containing colourings, flavourings or other additives (preservatives)
- citrus fruits.

All of these would be omitted from the diet totally, as would any other foods to which the individual has an obvious history of allergy.

A further elimination is also included, at first, of any foods which the person being treated is known to eat regularly (daily or more than five times a week).

When all of these are cut from the diet this leaves a very limited range of foods to be eaten for several weeks before the gradual reintroduction of excluded foods, one at a time.

This diet has been very successful in providing the clues as to which foods should ultimately be permanently excluded. Initially the total exclusion is for just a few weeks, with the gradual reintroduction of foods – one at a time – each new food being assessed for at least four or five days before the next is reintroduced, to see whether symptoms return.

If symptoms improve during the total elimination and if they return when a particular food is eaten again, it is once again eliminated for at least six months to allow the body to become desensitized to it.

## Skin Problems

If a food is reintroduced and produces symptoms, a period of four or five days is allowed before another food is reintroduced.

If such a strategy is tried it is important to make a careful note of any symptom patterns as the changes are made – both during elimination and especially during reintroduction.

### Method 2: Simple Elimination Diet

Choose just one of the 'suspicious' food groups mentioned in Method 1 above, and eliminate this from your diet for at least 10 days. If there is an improvement in your skin condition during the latter part of the 10 days, then reintroduce the food and eat it several times daily for a few days to see if this brings on any return or flare-up of symptoms. If so, eliminate the food from your diet. If there is no change when leaving it out and when reintroducing it, then just continue to eat it as normal. This method is not as efficient as that described as Method 1, but is easier to maintain.

### Method 3: The Oligoantigenic Diet

The oligoantigenic diet is derived from many years of research in the UK at the Great Ormond Street Hospital for Sick Children and at Addenbrooke Hospital, Cambridge.

The eating pattern, detailed below, has been found very helpful in identifying the allergens which can trigger eczema and other skin conditions (as well as recurrent ear infections, asthma, bedwetting, hyperactivity and bowel problems, especially in children).

The oligoantigenic diet is usually followed for up to three weeks while symptoms are evaluated. If symptoms vanish, then one or more of the foods being avoided may be to blame. Identification and subsequent avoidance of the culprit food(s) depends upon the symptom returning with the reintroduction (challenge) of the food.

Meats

- Allowed: lamb, turkey, rabbit, game (lean and cooked plainly)
- Forbidden: beef, chicken, pork, preserved meats, bacon, sausages

Fish

- Allowed: white fish (not if eczema present)
- Forbidden: all smoked fish, shellfish

Vegetables

- Allowed: all except those listed as forbidden, below Patients with bowel problems are asked to avoid beans, lentils, Brussels sprouts and cabbage as well

## Skin Problems

- Forbidden: potatoes, tomatoes, onions, soya and sweetcorn

### Fruit

- Allowed: bananas, peeled pears, pomegranates, paw-paw, mango
- Forbidden: all fruits except the five allowed ones

### Cereals

- Allowed: rice, sago, millet, buckwheat
- Forbidden: wheat, oats, rye, barley, corn

### Oils

- Allowed: sunflower, safflower, linseed, olive
- Forbidden: corn, soya, 'vegetable', nut (especially peanut)

### Dairy

- Allowed: none (Tomor and Vitasieg products are exceptions to this)
- Forbidden: cow's milk and all its products including yogurt, butter, most margarines; all goat, sheep and soya milk products, eggs

## Drinks

- Allowed: some herbal teas such as camomile; pure water
- Forbidden: tea, coffee, fruit squashes, citrus drinks, apple juice, alcohol, tap water, carbonated drinks

## Miscellaneous

- Allowed: sea salt
- Forbidden: yeast products, chocolate, preservatives, *all food additives*, herbs, spices, honey, sugar of any sort

To make sense of what is happening on any exclusion diet, professional advice is needed. Several (up to three) weeks on an oligoantigenic diet might dramatically improve a wide range of symptoms resulting from allergy. Identifying what those foods are requires patience and, usually, professional help as the slow reintroduction is carried out, much as in Method 1 outlined above.

### Method 4: Stone Age Diet

A basic ideal diet for anyone who is allergic to foods is known as a Stone Age Diet. This eliminates any food which has been introduced to the human diet since Stone Age times, including all dairy produce, grains, domesticated animal products and all processed foods, additives, preservatives, etc. This method has been used very successfully in Scandinavia for treating allergic skin complaints (and also asthma).

Foods which *can* be eaten include:

- almost all vegetables and fruits (apart from tropical and citrus fruits)
- game, lamb and fish (although many people are also sensitive to fish)
- For some people the restrictions during which gradual testing is undertaken may call for a basic 'pears and lamb' diet.

## Diet for Non-allergic Skin Problems

The following basic dietary rules should be adhered to by anyone who has skin problems or, for that matter, health problems of any kind.

- Avoid all refined carbohydrates – sugar or white flour products (cakes, sweets, pastries, pastas, bread made from anything other than wholemeal flour).
- Avoid all animal fats. This means cutting out milk other than skimmed milk, cheese other than low-fat cheese; all fat on meat (game is better because it

## Diet and Skin Problems

contains a different type of fat than that found in red meats, and is of lower fat content).
- Avoid butter and margarine as well as cream and ice-cream.
- Vegetable oils should be restricted to modest use of olive oil and/or sunflower oil.
- Yogurt is allowed if this is low fat and 'live' (containing the helpful *acidophilus* bacteria) with no additives.
- Avoid all chemicalized foods. This includes most canned goods and all processed foods which contain preservatives, colourings, flavourings, stabilizers, etc.
- Avoid fried food and roasts. These ways of cooking produce undesirable changes in fats.
- Avoid soft drinks, alcohol and vinegar. Coffee and tea should be taken in moderation only (no more than two cups per day unsugared).
- Avoid chocolate.
- Keep grain-based foods to a modest level (no more than three slices of wholemeal bread daily).

The eating pattern could be something like this:

- *Breakfast:* natural live yogurt; fresh fruit; a seed and nut (non-sugared) muesli (oats, freshly-milled nuts such as almond or hazel, seeds such as sunflower or pumpkin, sesame or linseed – all available from

health food stores). This mixture may be moistened with low-fat yogurt, apple juice or water and eaten with fruit. Wholemeal bread and yeast spread (if there is no Candida problem – *see page 109*); egg (if no allergy noted); herbal tea (camomile, etc.).
- *Snacks:* fresh fruit, seeds and nuts.
- *Lunch/Supper:* one of these should be a salad-based meal together with a rice (unpolished) dish, or baked potato, or wholemeal bread. For protein, cottage cheese or other low-fat cheese or fish. Dress salad with olive oil (cold-pressed) and lemon juice. Salads should be varied and contain different types of vegetables as available.
- *Main meal:* the other main meal should be a cooked protein meal. This could contain fish, poultry (avoid the fatty skin) or lean meat, or a vegetarian savoury made from lentils, nuts, beans, grains, etc. together with cooked vegetables.
- Desserts should be fruit.
- Recommended drinks include herbal teas, spring water and fruit juices.

Always chew food well and attempt to eat in a relaxed atmosphere, not when you're overtired or on edge. Never overeat and do not drink much whilst eating.

This pattern of eating, interspersed with periodic days of detoxification, will serve as a basis for recovery from skin and other health problems.

## Why Detoxification and Fasting Help to Produce Better Skin (and Overall Health)

Your mind-body defends itself against and copes with invading micro-organisms, toxic materials, changes in temperature, unpleasant situations and a bewildering variety of stresses and strains, of a mechanical (for example, posture), biochemical and emotional nature. For our entire lives we are in a state of adaptation, as this struggle to retain balance – equilibrium – continues.

Your body repairs itself, given the chance – broken bones mend, cuts heal and the vast majority of infections are dealt with efficiently and without symptoms. Even when symptoms appear they are often only evidence of the body doing its self-repair and self-healing work. Fever, inflammation, diarrhoea, vomiting and many skin complaints are all evidence of the immune and other repair systems of the body performing their survival tasks.

Many emotions such as anxiety and depression are only evidence of excessive degrees of perfectly normal emotions. It would be abnormal not to feel anxious in a situation of danger – however, an excessive amount of anxiety is not normal.

In just the same way, allergies are often evidence of an over-reaction on the part of the defence systems of the body to undesirable substances, to which some reaction is perfectly normal.

## Skin Problems

While physical symptoms are often unpleasant they are often lifesaving – think of the pain of an appendix about to burst – without it death would arrive silently. Without fever the body could not deal with invading microbes, viruses, parasites, etc. Without inflammatory processes, the repair of damaged tissues could not take place. Without the ability to purge ourselves rapidly of the danger (vomiting, diarrhoea, etc.) poisons could rapidly kill us ... and so on.

Many skin complaints are also forms of elimination, or may represent ways in which the body is dealing with something of a more chronic nature, perhaps bowel toxicity or an inefficient liver.

On a less dramatic scale we can see that a host of stress factors are making demands on our adaptation and repair processes all the time – both emotionally and biochemically, through toxic exposure, the relatively denatured quality of our food and the major emotional stresses of modern life. These multiple and complex demands can ultimately overwhelm our capacity to adapt – especially if they are interacting on a mind-body complex which has inherited imbalances and weaknesses from the start. A gradual decline in health therefore becomes inevitable, often signalled by the onset of what has been called 'vertical ill-health' in which we develop a range of minor symptoms which are not severe enough to send us to bed (horizontal ill-health) and which are seen as 'normal' because so

*Diet and Skin Problems*

many others have the same problems – ranging from digestive problems to minor skin complaints, headaches, disturbed sleep, aches and pains, etc.

## What's to Be Done about 'the Stress of Life'?

There are only three strategies which can offer a beneficial change to the inevitable decline in health caused by the biochemical, mechanical and emotional stressors impacting on your defence systems:

(a) You can try to *remove the causes* (eat better, exercise better, sleep better, relax more, etc.), so reducing the demands being made on the adaptive, repair and defence capabilities of the body.
(b) You can try to *improve the adaptive, repair and defence capabilities of the body* by methods which enhance immune and repair functions.
(c) You can *treat the symptoms* – either in a way which causes no new problems (the ideal) or in ways which mask symptoms and actually create new problems – which is bad medicine.

Examples of the last point are the use of anti-inflammatory drugs for arthritis, painkillers for a headache and antacid medication for indigestion – all of which can ease symptoms but do nothing to remove causes, and as a rule create 'side-effects' and therefore new problems for the body to deal with.

In summary we can try to reduce the stress load and/or improve our ability to handle it, or we can try to palliate the effects of our handling of the load – well or badly – or of course we can choose to do nothing and simply crumble under the onslaught.

## Natural Healing Objectives

Unlike the use of medication and many types of surgical intervention, which impose solutions or which make forced alterations to the situation, natural healing methods start by respecting the self-healing (homoeostatic) potentials of the body.

This is sometimes referred to as *vis medicatrix naturae* or the 'healing power of nature'. In some old texts it is called 'awakening the physician within', and in more scientific terminology as 'enhancing homoeostasis'.

Whatever words are used to describe such methods, they appear to work by allowing space, giving a healing opportunity and doing the opposite of forcing a solution, which might offer only short-term benefits.

Fasting sits at the centre of such approaches, along with relaxation and meditation methods, the use of relaxing hydrotherapy methods (such as the 'Epsom Salt bath' described on page 86; see also Chapter 7), the use of non-specific bodywork ('wellness massage' and aromatherapy relaxation methods, for example) and employment of techniques which have a

## Diet and Skin Problems

balancing, harmonizing, normalizing influence – including some herbal and acupuncture methods.

None of these methods, in itself, is 'curative', but all allow the body's healing potential to operate more efficiently because they offer the essential time, space and reduced demands which encourage normalization and recovery, irrespective of whatever is wrong.

This is not to say that such methods can produce absolute remedies in all cases, since in many instances pathology will have created so much change, so much damage, that the best that can be hoped for is that matters do not get worse, or that there is a marginal improvement. This is nevertheless an infinitely better outcome than a steady decline into ever more ill-health.

Natural healing approaches in general, and fasting in particular, can produce spectacularly beneficial results – a return to well-being, to vital, energetic, clear-headed, bright-eyed, clean-skinned wellness.

Trevor Salloum, ND, a famous American naturopath, describes the benefits of fasting:

> …decreased weight, clearer skin, increased elimination, tissue repair, decreased pain and inflammation, increased concentration, relaxation, plus spare time and savings in the cost of food. Perhaps the greatest benefit is the satisfaction that you are taking a major role in improving your health.

*Skin Problems*

## Detox for the Skin

To restore health in cases of chronic skin complaints, regular periods of inner cleansing are necessary. One day per week at least should be set aside for a 'raw food day', and at least once a month this should be turned into a fast day.

- On raw food days, only fruits, nuts and salads may be eaten as desired, but nothing cooked.
- On fast days, only liquids are consumed. It is important that at least 2 litres (4 pints) of liquid be consumed on such days. This should be spring water or diluted fruit juice (e.g. 50 per cent apple/ 50 per cent water). It is not necessary to stay in bed on fast days, but activity should be confined to gentle walks and a fair amount of time allowed for rest.
- On fast days the intake of supplements should be stopped, apart from *acidophilus* powder which should be continued at the normal rate.

## Monodiets

If you find fasting on liquids only too difficult, then eat one form of fruit only for the day's fast.

Grapes are an ideal choice and may be eaten, together with consumption of natural grape juice, to form a modified fast with great benefit. The one-day fast involves a 36-hour period, by starting on the evening prior to the fast and ending the morning after the fast. Eat a fruit and salad meal one evening, fast the next day and eat a fruit and yogurt breakfast the following morning.

## Supplements for Skin Problems

*(See also special notes on yeast-related problems later in this chapter.)*

The following supplements are recommended for all those afflicted by skin problems. The quantities stated are for adults and should be modified accordingly by body weight for children. Before embarking on any supplement regime, always check with your health care provider.

- Vitamin C – 1 to 2 g daily. The dose should be divided between morning and evening. The form of vitamin C should be one which also contains bioflavonoids. This will be stated on the container or packaging. People with psoriasis should not take more than 500 mg of vitamin C daily.
- Vitamin E – 200 to 400 iu daily
- Selenium – to be taken with vitamin E, 50 to 200 microgrammes (mcg) daily.
- Vitamin A – 20,000 to 50,000 iu daily (no more unless taken under supervision).

## Skin Problems

- Zinc – in the form of zinc orotate, 100 to 200 mg daily. This will provide 15 to 30 mg of actual zinc. Together with zinc, the B vitamin pyridoxine ($B_6$) is necessary – at least 50 mg daily is required.
- Chromium – as an orotate, 10 mg daily.
- Vitamin B complex – one strong source of B complex should be taken daily, containing not less than 50 mg each of the major B vitamins, such as niacin.
- EPA (eicosapentaenoic acid) – suitable for eczematous problems.
- *Lactobacillus acidophilus* and *Bifidobacteria* – ideally in powdered form. Dissolve and drink a quarter teaspoonful of each twice daily in a little lukewarm water away from meal times. Those sensitive to milk should take dairy-free forms; those not sensitive to milk may take these or a dairy-based *acidophilus* and *bifidus*. If powdered versions are not available, take a capsule – but never a tablet as the formation of this damages the sensitive bacteria organisms.
- Biotin – 500 mcg twice daily.
- Evening primrose oil or Flaxseed oil – 500 to 1,000 mg daily.
- Calcium – 500 to 1,000 mg daily.

## To Enhance Detoxification

- Cysteine – 1 to 2 g daily, together with vitamins $B_6$ and C (as above).
- Methionine – ½ to 1 g daily, away from meal times, with water.

## For Herpes

- Lysine – 300 to 1,200 mg daily, together with vitamin C.

## For All Inflammatory Conditions

- Quercetin – this bioflavonoid should be taken regularly by those with inflammatory lesions, 1 teaspoonful of powder three times daily is suggested, together with bromelain, 500 mg three times daily.

# Yeast (Candida albicans) and Skin Problems

The use of antibiotics and steroid medication (including the contraceptive Pill) can lead to the spread of yeasts in the intestinal tract and the body generally. These yeasts are normally controlled by 'friendly' bacteria, which are damaged by these types of medication.

## Skin Problems

The main yeast engaged in such activity is *Candida albicans*, best known for causing thrush. Candida is dangerous because of its ability to turn from a simple yeast into an aggressive mycelial fungus which puts down 'rootlets' (rhizomes) into the mucous membrane of the intestinal tract, so permitting undesirable toxins to move from the gut into the bloodstream, with the strong possibility of allergic and toxic reactions taking place as a result.

Among the many symptoms which have been catalogued in people affected in this way are a range of digestive symptoms (bloating, swings from diarrhoea to constipation and back), urinary tract infections, menstrual disturbances, fatigue, muscle aches, emotional disturbances, 'foggy' brain symptoms and, last but by no means least, a range of skin problems including acne and actual skin fungal problems such as ringworm and athlete's foot. The frequency with which such symptoms are suffered by people with a yeast overgrowth in the intestinal tract is enormous.

Laboratory tests to 'prove' yeast involvement are commonly inaccurate, mainly because almost everyone on the planet has some yeast living in their digestive tract and simply finding it there does not help to determine just how widespread its presence is.

Diagnosis by symptoms is more accurate and if an anti-Candida programme makes the symptoms vanish or improve greatly, this confirms the diagnosis.

*Diet and Skin Problems*

One of the most useful tests involves a sugar-loading test – a sample of blood is taken, then 100 g of sugar are consumed on an empty stomach, then another sample of blood is taken one hour later. This test assesses the level of alcohol in the blood before and after the sugar intake, because yeast – and some bacteria – can turn sugar into alcohol rapidly in the intestines.

## When to Suspect Candida

Candida may prove to be a factor in your health or skin problems if after examining the lists below you find that one item or more from each section applies in your case.

(a) Have you:
   a history of long-term antibiotic usage (one long period of taking them – more than two months – or more than four courses in any one year)? This would have damaged the normal flora and allowed the always present yeast to spread.
   ever taken a course of tetracycline (or any other antibiotic) to treat acne for more than one month?
   ever taken the contraceptive pill for more than two years consistently?
   been pregnant more than twice?
(b) And, do you (or have you):
   suffered from persistent prostatitis or vaginitis?
   had ringworm or athlete's foot?

had cravings for sugar or bread or alcohol?
(c) And are you currently suffering from:
fatigue?
digestive bloating or 'irritable bowel'?
'foggy brain' (short-term memory difficulties, concentration problems)?
widespread muscular aches and pains?
thrush?
loss of sexual interest?
premenstrual tension?

If you consider that you may have a Candida overgrowth, you may want to consult an expert who deals with such problems, or to read more about it (see my book *Candida Albicans – Could Yeast Be Your Problem?*, Thorsons, 1995).

**The skin conditions which are likely to be associated with Candida, apart from ringworm, fungal nail problems and athlete's foot, are chronic acne and psoriasis. These conditions may appear to be worse for the first few weeks of an anti-Candida diet (see below).**

The recommendations given here represent an absolute minimum strategy which should be carried out for not less than three months. Ideally this should be under the supervision of a suitably trained nutritional expert (naturopath, medical herbalist, clinical ecologist, nutritional counsellor, dietitian, etc.).

## Three-month Basic Anti-Candida Strategy

1. Caprylic acid (coconut plant extract) – 1 capsule with each meal (that is, three times a day). Acts as an antifungal.
2. Biotin – 500 mcg twice a day. This B vitamin helps to control the yeast's tendency to alter to a more aggressive form.
3. High-potency garlic – 1 capsule with each meal (three times a day). Antifungal, antibiotic.
4. Either any of the following three herbs, individually or in combination:
   *Hydrastis canandensis* (Goldenseal)
   *Berberis vulgaris* (Barberry) and/or
   *Echinacea angustifolia* (Purple Coneflower)
   – three times daily as an antifungal immune-enhancing support
   and/or
   Pau D'arco tea – three to four times daily.
   These herbs should be obtained from a reputable herbal supplier or health food store and used according to the instructions on the pack.

## Encouraging Repopulation of Intestinal Flora

5. High-quality *acidophilus* and *Bifidobacteria* (powder or capsule form) – between meals (three times

*Skin Problems*

daily), either a capsule of each, or a quarter teaspoon of the powdered versions of each.
6 General nutritional support is useful – taking a well-formulated, yeast-free, hypoallergenic, multivitamin/ multimineral to provide at least the recommended daily allowance of the major nutrients.

## Dietary Suggestions for Candida

- Chew well/eat slowly/try not to drink much with meals.
- Eat three small main meals daily as well as two snack meals where possible (no sugar-rich food), or take 3 to 5 grams of full-spectrum amino acid complex between main meals, twice daily.
- Include in the diet as much ginger, cinnamon and garlic (as well as other aromatic herbs such as oregano) as possible – all are antifungal and most also aid digestive processes.
- To assist with bowel function, regularly (daily, same time of day) take at least 1 tablespoonful of linseed. Swallow with water, unchewed to provide a soft fibre to assist intestinal emptying.
- **Avoid as far as possible all refined sugars** and for the first few weeks avoid very sweet fruit as well (melon, sweet grapes). Avoid aged cheeses, dried fruits and any food obviously derived from or

*Diet and Skin Problems*

containing yeast (in case of sensitization).
- Avoid caffeine (coffee, tea, chocolate, cola, etc.) as this produces a sugar release which is not desirable where yeast has proliferated.
- Avoid alcohol.
- If possible avoid all yeast-based foods – including bread and anything that contains yeast in its manufacture or which might contain mould.

You may feel off-colour for the first week of such a programme as yeast 'die-off' takes place.

Note:
Many other antifungal substances are available and may be more effective in certain cases than the suggestions above, which are however usually beneficial if the programme is maintained for several months.

## Sources

Almost all the supplements and most of the herbs mentioned in this book are now widely available from better health food stores and many pharmacies.

The Nutri Centre (7 Park Crescent, London W1 0171–436 5122) stocks all of the recommended nutrients and herbs and will supply to personal shoppers as well as by mail order (credit card required).

# 9
# Stress and the Skin

The instant result on the skin of emotional reactions is self-evident. We blush, flush and sweat in response to a variety of situations in completely unique ways. No two people will be the same in this respect.

Other factors such as nutritional status, hormonal balance, inherited tendencies, etc. will decide in which of us hormonal, secretory, neurological and circulatory influences, mediated by the mind's response to stress and anxiety, will result in long-term problems in the skin. The skin is very much influenced by our state of mind as well as certain other factors. In some people it is the primary factor.

Even in allergic conditions it can be shown that removal of stress and anxiety reduces the response of the person to the allergen, and sometimes removes the allergy altogether. This is because it is not the substance which is causing the problem, but rather the way the person is reacting to that substance which matters. That same element, whether it is pollen or house dust, or a chemical of some sort, will produce no reaction in most people, which proves that it is not the culprit. The imbalances in our bodies which allow it to provoke eczema, asthma or urticaria, are the culprits. And to a large extent such underlying factors are mind-controlled.

In severe skin conditions such as scleroderma, where the entire skin surface becomes hardened and calcified, it has been shown that the mind's powers are operating. One classic case demonstrated that a patient with scleroderma was hypnotized and told to allow the skin to soften and return to normal. Precisely that happened, and it was a permanent improvement.

Trials in the US have shown that teaching teenagers basic relaxation techniques allows them to rid their faces and bodies of chronic acne.

The mind and the skin are closely interconnected, which is not to say that we can ignore the nutritional and hygienic factors already outlined. The truth is that the body expresses diseases and dysfunction in so many ways and the causes are multiple. No one element on its own will result in the particular disease, on the skin or elsewhere. It requires that combination of inherited tendencies, dietary imbalances (toxicities and deficiencies) as well as mental/emotional factors before problems unique to the individual will manifest themselves.

This is why the apparent same causative factors produce very different problems in people with quite different dietary and environmental backgrounds.

Worry, grief, anxiety and general stress and emotional strain will influence the hormonal and neurological systems of the body and also the all-important digestive functions. The answer to this element of mind-related factors is to learn and practise methods which reduce anxiety and stress. This calls for a programme of action which is too lengthy to more than outline in this book.

Try to avoid stress-inducing situations and habits and take regular practice in relaxation techniques. In this way the element of easy arousal and undesirable reaction will gradually drop away. The benefits will be reflected in the skin, as well as in other body systems, for example blood pressure and digestion.

## Relaxation Exercises

Relaxation exercises are most important in helping to bring stress down to acceptable levels. One, at least, of the following should be employed each day for not less than 10 minutes, and if blood-pressure problems are evident, then twice daily is suggested. These should be done at a different time from the breathing exercises,

## Stress and the Skin

and always when there is no likelihood of being disturbed. Find a quiet room and settle into a chair, or recline on a couch, or on the floor.

## Breathing and Repeated Sound Technique

Sit or lie in a comfortable position in a suitable place. Close your eyes and encourage a sense of heaviness and stillness. Focus your attention on the body, area by area, briefly, in order to assess each one for obvious tension. Start with the feet and pass on to the lower legs, thighs, hips, buttocks, abdomen, lower back, chest, shoulders, neck, face, arms and hands. Do not overlook the eyes and jaw muscles. Many people screw up the eye muscles or clench the jaw habitually. If this is one of your traits, then pay particular attention to releasing these areas prior to continuing with the exercise.

This should only be a brief survey, not lasting for more than a few seconds in each region. As each area is visualized, any obvious tension should be released. If you are not sure whether a muscle or area is relaxed, tense it for a few seconds and then let it go. This brief but effective progressive muscular relaxation, area by area, prepares you for the exercise proper. It is worth emphasizing that relaxation is a passive act. You cannot 'try' to relax, for this is a contradiction in terms. Relaxation is a letting go, a switch-off, which ideally involves no effort. Suggesting that dubious areas be

## Skin Problems

tensed prior to 'letting go' is only to help to imprint on the mind the contrast between the two states. In this way, a gradual awareness will develop, enabling you to sense tension as it arises and, most importantly, to release it. (This is the basis of progressive muscular relaxation methods.)

For the purpose of this exercise the method outlined above is all that is required as preparation for the following breathing exercise.

Having spent a minute or, at most, two, in 'letting go' the obvious areas of tension in the musculature of the body, begin to breathe in and out through the nose. Passively pay attention to your breathing and, as you breathe out, say silently and slowly to yourself any one-syllable word. Breathe in and out at any comfortable speed; there need be no rush, nor is there any need to make the breathing particularly slow. The rhythm should be as natural and unforced as possible, not particularly deep or unusually shallow.

You may well find that the rhythm will alter from time to time, or that periodically you will let out a very deep breath or sigh. Just let it happen, do not attempt to control the rhythm or depth of the respiration – simply use it to time the repetitive, slow enunciation of a word or sound. Many people use the word 'one' for this purpose, but any short word will do. Remember it should be said as you breathe out. This should continue for about 10 minutes.

## Stress and the Skin

A feeling of stillness and calm should eventually be felt. In some cases a sense of happiness and deep relaxation is quickly achieved. In others there is only a gradual sense of being less stressed. In all cases where this type of exercise is performed as described, positive physiological changes will take place, irrespective of subjective feelings. In other words, there is a degree of stress-reduction, whether or not you sense it from the outset.

Many people expect immediate, obvious changes. If disappointed in this expectation, they may abandon the discipline involved in the regular performance of these exercises. This is sad and a waste, for it has been positively established that the benefits of the exercises often begin long before there is any awareness of improvement.

The repetition of the chosen word may well be interrupted periodically by intrusive thoughts. When this happens, do not feel irritated, simply resume the use of the word to coincide with exhalation. Each individual will reap the benefits of this exercise at his or her own pace.

After about 10 minutes of this exercise, stop repeating the word and simply allow the mind the luxury of doing nothing. Allow it to linger in the still, peaceful state to which you have drifted. Initially with the eyes closed and later with them open, spend at least two minutes in this state of inactivity. Slowly get up and resume your normal activities. (It is unwise to get up too quickly as over-oxygenation may result in transient giddiness).

## Progressive Muscular Relaxation

This method involves the systematic, conscious relaxation of all the body areas in sequence. The position for this exercise should be reclining – either on the floor or on a recliner-type chair. Ideally, there should be no distracting sounds and the clothing worn should not constrict in any way. (A few cycles of deep breathing should precede the exercise.)

Starting with the feet, try to sense or feel that the muscles of the area are not actively tense. Then deliberately tighten them, curling the toes under and holding the tension for five to ten seconds. Then tense the muscles even more strongly for a further few seconds before letting all the tension go and sensing the wonderful feeling of release. Try to register consciously what this feels like, especially in comparison with the tense state in which you have been holding them. Progress to the calf muscles and exercise them in the same way. First sense the state the muscles are in, then tense them, hold the position, and then tense them even more before letting go. Positively register the sense of release. In doing this to the leg muscles, there is a slight danger of inducing cramp. If this occurs stop testing that area immediately and move on to the next.

After the calf muscles, go on to exercise the knees, then the upper leg, thigh muscles, the buttocks, the lower and upper back, the abdomen, the chest, the shoulders, the arms and hands, and then the neck, head and face. The precise sequence is irrelevant, as long as all these areas are 'treated' to the tensing, the extra tensing, and then the release.

Some areas need extra attention in this respect. The abdominal region is a good example. The tensing of these muscles can be achieved in either contraction (i.e. a pulling in of the muscles), or by stretching (i.e. a pushing outwards of the muscles). The variation in tensing method is applicable to many of the body's muscles. Indeed, at different times it is a good idea to vary the pattern, and instead of, for example, contracting and tensing a muscle group, try to stretch and tense them to their limit. This is especially useful in the muscles of the face, particularly in the mouth and eye region. Individual attention to these is important. On one occasion it would be desirable, for example, for the 'tensing' of the mouth muscles to take the form of holding the mouth open as wide as possible, with the lips tense during this phase. On a subsequent occasion the 'tensing' could be a tight-pursed pressing together of the lips. If there is time available, both methods of tensing can be employed during the same exercise, especially in the areas you know to be very tense. The muscles controlling the jaw, eyes, mouth, tongue and neck are particularly important, as are the abdominal muscles, since much emotional tension is reflected in these regions and release and relaxation often has profound effects.

There are between 20 and 25 of these 'areas', depending upon how you go about interpreting the guidelines given above; each should involve at least five to 10 seconds of 'letting go' and of passively sensing that feeling. Thus, eight to 10 minutes should suffice for the successful completion of this whole technique. This should be followed by several minutes of an unhurried return to a feeling of warm, relaxed tranquillity. Focus the mind on the whole body. Try to sense it as heavy and content, free of tension or effort. This might be enhanced by a few cycles of deep breathing. Stretch out like a cat, and then resume your normal activities.

## Autogenic Exercises

True autogenic exercises need to be taught by a special teacher or practitioner well versed in this excellent system. The modified method outlined below is based on the work of the pioneer in this field, Dr H. Schultz. The distinction between a relaxation exercise and a meditation technique is blurred at all times, but never more so than in autogenic methods, which are a blend of the two. At least 15 and ideally 20 minutes should be given to the performance of this method. At another

## Stress and the Skin

time of the day this, or another relaxation method, should also be performed again. This routine should become a welcome, eagerly anticipated oasis of calm and peace in the daily programme. Stress-proofing without such periods of 'switching off' is unlikely to be successfully achieved.

A reclining position should be adopted, with the eyes closed. External, distracting sounds should be minimized. The exercises involve the use of specific, verbalized messages to focus awareness on a particular area. No effort is involved, but simply a passive concentration on any sensations or emotions which may result from each message. Imagination or auto-suggestion has been found to have definite physiological effects. By combining a sequence of autogenic (i.e. self-generated) instructions, with the passive, focused aspect of meditation techniques, a powerful method of self-help has been created.

The exercise starts with a general thought, such as 'I am relaxed and at peace with myself.' Begin to breathe deeply in and out. Feel the light movement of the diaphragm and feel calm.

### Stage I

The mind should focus on the area of the body to which the thought is directed. Start by silently verbalizing 'My right arm is heavy.' Think of the image of the right arm. Visualize it completely relaxed, and resting on its support (the floor, arm of the chair, etc.). Dissociate it from the body and from will-power. See the limp, detached arm as being heavy, having weight. After a few seconds the phrase should be repeated. This should be done a number of times before proceeding to the right leg, left leg, left arm, neck, shoulders and back. At each area, try to sense heaviness and maintain a passive feeling in the process.

## Stage II

Again begin with the right arm, concentrating on it as you silently verbalize 'My right arm is warm.' Repeat this and pause to sense warmth in the arm or hand. Repeat this several times. The pause should be unhurried. To encourage this feeling of warmth it may be useful to imagine that the sun's rays are shining onto the back of the hand warming it. The sensation of warmth spreads from there to the whole arm.

Proceed through all areas of the body, pausing for some seconds at each to assess sensations which may become apparent. Such changes as occur cannot be controlled, but will happen when the mind is in a passive, receptive state. This exercise increases the peripheral flow of blood, and relaxes the muscles controlling the blood-vessels. It is possible to increase measurably the temperature of an area of the body using these simple methods.

## Stage III

The phrase 'I am alert and refreshed' ends the exercise. Breathe deeply, stretch, and continue the day's activities.

During Stages I and II, the time spent in each area should not be less than about half a minute; it is however quite permissible to spend two or three minutes focusing on any one part, especially if the desired sensation of heaviness or warmth is achieved.

It will probably be found that the desired sensation is more easily sensed in one stage than another, and that some areas seem more 'responsive' than others. This is normal. It is also quite normal for there to be no subjective appreciation of any of the verbalized sensations. Do not worry about this. Even if nothing at all is sensed for some considerable time, possibly months, there is a great deal actually taking place within the body as a result of the whole exercise. Persistence, patience and a total lack of urgency is all that is necessary for this method to lead to a decrease in muscular tension and a sense of calm and well-being. A side-effect of this particular method is frequently experienced in terms of much improved peripheral circulation, i.e. an end to cold hands and feet.

## Exercise

Regular aerobic exercise (not less than 30 minutes, three times weekly) is stress-reducing and also assists in skin function. It can be applied by anyone in whatever state of unfitness. Walking or more active exercise patterns can be employed to achieve the desired effects of enhancement of cardio-vascular efficiency, stress-reduction and skin function.

# Summary

There are many causes of skin problems and we must deal with all of them. We must reform our eating habits as discussed and support the self-healing functions of the body by nutrient supplementation.

There are a number of simple and useful direct approaches involving water, clay and other substances (e.g. aloe vera) which can be safely employed in local treatment.

Hygiene of the body and skin is a key element in skin health, involving the use of skin friction, sun and air baths. The health of the bowel is fundamental to good skin health and also calls for dietary assistance where dysfunction exists.

Finally, the element of the mind must be brought into the healing process – reduction in stress, lifestyle (adequate exercise and rest) and also specific relaxation exercises. Mental imagery helps to visualize a healthy body covered by a healthy skin.

All this takes patience and time, because it is attempting to reverse processes which may have been operating for a long time. Self-help means attention to the needs of the whole person, not just the local disturbance. Local treatment is never an end in itself, but rather a temporary measure which is carried out whilst underlying causes are being dealt with. Self-healing works but is not necessarily as quick as the apparent dramatic results of drugs which, however, are usually only masking the condition and which almost always produce side-effects. A healthy body and a healthy skin will result from the programme outlined in this book. All it takes is effort.

# Index

abcesses 88
acidophilus *see Lactobacillus acidophilus*
acne 13, 42, 43, 65–74, 112
*acne conglobata* 65–6
*acne vulgaris* 65
acupressure 11
acupuncture 11, 104
Addison's disease 37
aerobic exercise 33, 128
ageing, of skin 20, 26, 30
air baths 31–2, 128
alcohol 34, 40
allergic rhinitis 47
allergies 101, 116–17
*see also* food allergies
aloe vera juice 47, 52, 82, 88
aloe vera ointment 52

amino acids 61, 80, 82
anaemia 36
anti-Candida diet 112–15
antibiotics:
　for acne 71–2
　effects 37, 109
antiperspirants 14, 33
antiseptics 47
anxiety 52, 101
aplastic anaemia 38
arginine 80
argyria 37
aromatherapy massage 104
arrectores pilorum muscle 10
asthma 47
athlete's foot 43, 111, 112
atopic dermatitis 43–53
atopic eczema 41, 45–6, 47, 49–50

## Index

autogenic exercises 124–7
autographism 38
axillary hidradenitis 42

bacteria:
   activity on skin 14
   infections 42
   penetration of 12
   and ultraviolet light 31
basal layer cells 9, 10
bathing 33–4, 52, 86–7
*Berberine (Berberis vulgaris)* 62, 113
Bifidobacteria 61, 108, 113–14
bioflavenoids 49, 107
biotin 78, 108, 113
blackheads 65
blemishes 4
blood blisters 37
blood diseases 38
blood sugar 16
blood vessels 9, 12, 18
bluish skin colour 36–7
body fluid level, control 4
boils 42, 88
bowel health 50–1, 61, 82, 128
breathing and repeated sound relaxation technique 119–22
bromelain 49, 60, 83, 109
bronze-like skin discoloration 37
brownish skin colour 37

bubble baths 47
burns 88–9

calcium 30, 63, 108
calendula products 70
camomile lotion 28
cancer 38
   *see also* skin cancer
Candida albicans 51, 71, 109–15
capillaries, fragile 38
caprylic acid 113
carbohydrates, refined 73
   study 91
carbuncles 42
carotinaemia 36
causes 103, 118
cells, in basal layer 9, 10
cerebrospinal meningitis 38
chemicals:
   exposure to, and acne 67
   penetration of 12
Cheraskin, Prof E. 90–1
cholesterol 36
chromium 73, 108
clay *see* green clay
cleansing function 3–4
cleansing method, for acne 70–1
clothing 32–3
cold compresses 87
cold sores 79
colds 32, 33
colour, of skin 5, 35–8
compresses 4, 87–8

131

## Skin Problems

contact dermatitis 42
contraceptive pill 68, 109
corium 9
cosmetics, and acne 68–9
cradle cap 46
cuticle 10
cyanosis 36–7
cysteine 61, 109

dandruff 77, 79
Dead Sea products 57
deodorants 14, 31
depression 101
dermatitis 42
dermatitis herpetiformis 43, 75
dermatographism 38
detergents 47
detoxification 61, 64, 106–7, 109
diabetes 36
diagnosis aid 5, 29, 35–40
diet 90–115
diets:
    for acne 72–4
    anti-Candida 112–15
    elimination 47, 53, 75, 92–8
    monodiets 106–7
    for non-allergic skin problems 98–100
    oligoantigenic 94–7
    pears and lamb 98
    for psoriasis 59–64
    rotation 53
    Stone Age 97–8
discoid eczema 41, 46

discoid lupus erythematosus 41
dry skin 14

ear wax 14
ecchymoses 37
*Echinacea* 62, 113
eczema 43–53
    types 41–2
eicosapentanoic acid (EPA) 49, 63, 82, 108
elasticity 30
elimination diets 47, 53, 75, 92–8
elimination function 3–4, 14, 19–20, 32–3, 102
epidermis 9–10
epithelium 10
Epsom salts 57, 87
erythema multiforme 42, 75–6
erythema nodosum 42
erythemato-squamous dermatopathies 41
essential fatty acids 34, 49, 50
evaporation compresses 87
evening primrose oil 50, 63, 64, 82, 108
exercise, aerobic 33, 128
exfoliation 31
exogenous eczema 44

face, avoid tan on 25
fasting 104–7
fat, subcutaneous 9, 34
fats, saturated 34, 73

## Index

feet:
    chronic eczema 41
    cold, improvement 127
fever 19
fibre 64
fish oil 63
flax seed oil 63, 78, 108
food, processed 34
food allergies 47–9, 53, 64
    risk foods 92–3
free radicals 39
fungal diseases 14, 41
furuncles 42

garlic 81, 113
gluten sensitivity 75
Goldenseal 60, 61–2, 113
green clay 52, 82, 83, 84–6
use for acne 70–1
grey-blue skin colour 37

haemochromatosis 37
hair follicles 9, 10, 13
hands:
    chronic eczema 41
    cold, improvement 127
health, decline 102–5
herbal medicine 104
herpes infections 42, 76, 79–80, 109
histamines 49, 50
homoeostasis 15–17
hormone activity:
    and sweating 14, 18
    and teenage acne 43, 66–7
    and women's acne 68

hormone creams 46
hot fomentations 88
*Hydrastis canadensis* see Goldenseal
hydrotherapy 11, 15, 57, 83, 86–8, 104

icthyosis 35
illness, effects 5
immune system 49, 61, 101
impetigo 42
infections 42
inflammation 83
intestinal flora, repopulation 113–14
iodine, and acne 73
irritants 4, 45, 47, 53
itching 45–6
    easing 4, 47, 51–2

jaundice 36

keratin 12
kidney disease 38
kinins 50
Kligman, Prof Albert 21, 24–5

*Lactobacillus acidophilus* 50, 61, 82, 108, 113–14
leukemia 38
lice 43
lichen planus 41
lichenification 43, 45–6
lipids 14
liver disease 38

## Skin Problems

lupus erythematosus 41
lymphatic structures 9, 14
lysine 80

massage 11, 104
meditation 104
melanin 21
methionine 61, 109
milk, allergy to 48
monodiets 106–7
multivitamins and minerals 114
mummular (discoid) eczema 41, 46
muscular relaxation 122–4
myxoedema 35
nails, fungal problems 112
natural healing 104–15
nerve endings 11–12
neutral baths 11–12, 104
nodules, on skin 23, 36
non-soap cleansers 47
nutritional supplements 49–51, 107–9, 113–14, 128

oatmeal baths 87
oedema 35
oligoantigenic diet 94–7
orange skin colour 36
oregano oil 60, 62
organ, skin as 4–5, 6
oxygen starvation 36–7

pain 11
paleness 35–6

papillae 9
papules, reddish 37
para amino benzoic acid (PABA) 75
parasites 43
patch testing 45
Pau d'arco tea 113
pears and lamb diet 98
pemphigus vulgaris 43
pernicious anaemia 36
petechiae 37–8
petrolatum gels 24–5
photoallergic eczema 44
photodermatosis 26–8
photosensitivity 26–8
phototoxic eczema 44
pityriasis rosea 41
polycythaemia vera 36
pores, blocked 14
potassium iodide 75–6
progressive muscular relaxation 122–4
*Propionibacterium acnes* 65
protein 73
  digestion, and psoriasis 59, 60
proteolytic enzymes 60
psoriasis 41, 52, 54–64, 88
  and Candida 112
puberty 66
purpurea 37–8

quercetin 49, 63, 83, 109

raw food days 106
reddening 36

# Index

reddish-purple skin colour 36
relaxation 104
  exercises 52, 118–27
repair processes, promoting 103–15
*Rhus tox* 80
ringworm 43, 81, 111, 112
rosacea 43, 81
rose spots 38
rotation diets 53

Salloum, Trevor 105
salt baths 57, 87
sarsaparilla 60
scabies 43
scarlet fever 36
scars 88–9
Schultz, Dr H. 124
scleroderma 35
sebaceous glands 9, 10, 13, 43
seborrhoeic dermatitis 76–9
seborrhoeic eczema 41, 46
sebum 9, 10, 13, 14, 65
selenium 49, 63, 74, 107
self-healing 2–3, 6–7, 101, 129
sense organ function 11–12
showers 33–4
silver salt poisoning 37
silymarin (milk thistle) 61
skin cancer 20
  risk factors 21–3
skin friction 33, 86, 128

skin-care routines, for acne 70–1
smoking 34, 39–40
soaps 33–4, 47
solar elastosis 26
SPF numbers 23–4
spider naevi 38
spots 66
  picking/squeezing 67
stasis eczema 41
steroid drugs 109
  topical 46
Stone Age diet 97–8
stress 52, 102–4
  and acne 74
  and emotional factors 116–18, 128–9
structure, of skin 8–15
subcutaneous fat 9, 34
sugar, in diet 73, 91
sulphonamides, effects 37
sulphur 61, 70
sun exposure 128
  for acne 70, 72
  for psoriasis 64
  unwelcome effects 20, 21–8, 36
sun, protection from:
  avoidance actions 23
  lotions/creams 23–4, 25
sunblocks 24, 25
sunscreens 23–4, 25
supplements *see* nutritional supplements
sweat 14, 19
  acidity 12

## Skin Problems

excessive 17
sweat glands 9, 10, 13–14, 17, 18
Swedish Bitters 60
sycosis barbae 42, 81–2
symptoms, treating 4, 103
syphilis, secondary 41
tea tree oil products 69, 70, 79
teenage acne 66–7
temperature control 4, 13, 15, 17–19
thickness, of skin 12
thyroid conditions 35, 51
tuberculosis 35, 38
ultraviolet light:
    lamps, use 70
    and psoriasis 56
    from sun 20, 21, 23–5
urticaria 42
Vaseline 24
verrucae 42
virus infections 42
vitamin A 34, 82, 107
    in acne treatment 71, 73
    for eczema 49
    for psoriasis 60, 63
vitamin BU6u 63, 78, 108, 109
vitamin B complex 34, 49, 78, 108
vitamin C 34, 82, 91, 107, 109

for herpes 80
and psoriasis 63–4, 107
vitamin D 30–1
vitamin deficiencies 38
vitamin E 82, 107
    for acne 74
    for burns and scars 88–9
    for eczema 49
    for psoriasis 62, 63
vitamin K 38
warts 23, 42
washing 31, 67
water 82
weals, raised 42
weeping eczema 45
weight loss 35
witch's marks 38
women, and acne 68–9
wrinkles 26, 39

yeast problems *see* Candida albicans
yellowish skin colour 36

zinc 34, 78, 82, 108
    for acne 73, 74
    for eczema 49
    for psoriasis 62, 63
zinc orotate 63, 108
zinc oxide cream or lotion 51, 64
zinc sulphate solution 76